CW01648461

Heart Healthy Diet

Paleolithic and Grain Free Recipes to Promote Better Health

Valerie Lewis

Table of Contents

Heart Healthy Diets Introduction

Enjoy a Heart-Healthy Diet along with Weight Loss

Go heart healthy and lose weight with the Paleolithic Diet and Grain Free Recipes. Heart disease is the number one killer in the nation, but by feeding your body properly, you can overcome. You will find abundant food choices, enjoy excellent health benefits, and lost weight. Two cookbooks in one, the first section teaches you how the Paleolithic Diet has been bringing longer, more productive lives to people for millions of years. The second section, Grain Free Recipes, will show you how there are alternatives to gluten-laced breads and pastas. This book was written to present conservative and rational choices to better diets and better health. Called the Paleolithic Diet, or Cave Man Diet, by some, this diet doesn't constrict the amount of calories that your body needs to stay healthy, but merely, goes back to the basics of healthy food.

Sugar, starch, bread and dairy products are considered to be villains in many strict diets, causing you to crave certain unhealthy foods. After awhile, your weakness kicks in and out the window, goes the diet. The Paleolithic Diet offers choices through amazingly simple menus that are delicious and filling. New products have been introduced that mimic flour, sugar and milk, making the switch, almost easy. Not to mislead, there are certain foods that are not recommended, like whole milk, white bread, or cream-filled rolls. These are the types of foods that raised havoc on your body in the first place.

Read how a low-sugar, low-salt, dairy-free and high protein diet can begin to address the problems of strokes, heart disease, diabetes, and other life-threatening illnesses. Processed foods, such as cold cuts, canned vegetables and meats, and imitation flavored items should also be avoided. They are treated with chemicals that were never intended for human consumption. The fact that they have a long shelf life, does not make them nutritional.

Snacks are one of the hardest foodstuffs to give up when starting a diet, but they don't have to be. Smoothies, granola bars and fruit muffins can be satisfying and healthy, too. If you thought that granola bars could only be found at the market, you were wrong. Learn how to make your own treats and create your own variations for different flavors. They will be more flavorful and you'll soon have the whole family hooked on them.

The Entree recipes will make you wonder what the difference is in what you are now eating and what these dishes contain. They are flavorful, delicious and high in vitamins and nutrients. The difference is in the products that are used during preparation. Try Green Chili Turkey Burgers, that use chilies and cilantro for flavoring, or Chicken with Cherries and Kale, that is not only tangy and fragrant, but beautiful, as well. These are just a couple of the examples of how eating healthy can be a treat each day, by using interesting recipes.

Breakfast can be an eye-opening experience with eggs, Canadian bacon and muffins made with raisins, almonds and cinnamon. While you will find no gluten-laced bread with the Paleolithic Diet, there are other ways to achieve breads by using alternative products. This recipe, in particular, uses almond flour and flax meal, in the place of white flour. Other unique recipes for desserts will also surprise you with a great natural taste. Foods will begin to taste richer and fuller when natural ingredients are used, as opposed to processed products.

Several medical experts have claimed that gluten can lead to feeling tired or anxious. Imagine all of the doctor appointments you have made over the years from just these two symptoms. Other, more serious problems can include digestive problems, high blood pressure, poor muscle tissue, high percentage of body fat, depression, and poor circulation in arteries. Any one of these diagnoses can lead to heart failure, and many times, does just that.

Gluten is not just an ingredient that is found in white bread. Wheat, bran, barley, bulgur, orzo, semolina and farina, are all types of grain that can be found in breads or pasta. This means that items such as cake, pie, muffins, pizza, tortillas and bagels can also carry this ingredient. But it doesn't stop there. Canned soup, potato chips, dressing, bouillon cubes, and a host of other items may use gluten to form a nice texture. Every recipe found in this cook book is gluten-free but always check the labels before purchasing goods from the store.

Deciding to try the Paleolithic Diet, along with Grain Free Recipes is not just for losing a few extra pounds or to protect your heart, as you approach middle age. Many people, around the world, have been following this way of life for thousands of years. Getting back to basics is the objective, provided by this book. If you are new to Paleolithic and Gluten-free dieting, you will find a meal planner that offers suggestions in getting started. There is a bit of prep work that will be required, such as checking all labels to see if products are gluten-free, buying fresh fruit and vegetables, as opposed to canned, and making the time to prep and cook. Most Americans have discovered, that quick is not always best. This is your health and future at stake. If you have kids, guide them toward naturals foods as opposed to chips, candy and soft drinks.

Use the information and recipes in this book as a guide for starting a healthier life. You could possibly head off sickness and disease, improve your mental clarity, and feel like enjoying activities. With the right exercise and a sensible diet, you could have many quality years to look forward to. The Paleolithic diet has changed many lives, for the better, by removing additives, preservatives, too much sugar, too much fat, dairy products, and gluten-laced breads, that can damage the intestinal lining, increase blood pressure and much, much more. The facts are clear and this book will make a great reference for future use. Make the time it takes to add years to your life, get started, and never look back.

Section 1: Paleolithic Cookbook Introduction

What is the Paleolithic Diet?

Also known as the caveman diet and the Stone Age diet, the Paleolithic diet is a diet which is low in sugar, low in sodium, largely dairy free and relatively high in protein. It's a diet based on the foods which would have been available to our pre-agrarian Neolithic ancestors. The Paleolithic diet isn't a carb-free or low carb diet, per se, but it is free of grains, with carbohydrates coming from fresh vegetables and fruits rather than grains.

This is also a diet which steers clear of processed foods, at least for the most part – and any processed foods included in the diet are as minimally changed from their natural state as possible. While you obviously don't have to hunt or gather your own ingredients (and to be honest, the diet does include many vegetables which weren't really developed until we started to settle down in agrarian communities), the idea is to avoid the modern processed foods which can wreak havoc on your health.

Better health is really the main goal of the diet and while it isn't actually geared towards weight loss, many people who adopt the Paleolithic diet do indeed experience weight loss, especially when combined with regular exercise. It really comes down to common sense for the most part. The paleolithic diet is rich in natural, fresh foods – in short, the kind of food which we know that we should be eating in the first place.

The recipes in this book are made using these ingredients: fresh produce, meat and nuts are the major players in these Paleolithic diet recipes. Following this diet will require a little bit of adjustment on your part and a little more time in the kitchen, at least until you get the hang of things – but once you start enjoying the health benefits of the Paleolithic diet, we think you'll agree it's a change well worth making. From main dishes to salads, soups to desserts and breakfast and brunch, these recipes cover all of the basics – so without further ado, let's get cooking, paleolithic style!

Entrees

Roasted Turkey with Balsamic Glaze and Apples

Number of servings: 8 – 10

Ingredients:

1 medium-sized turkey (10 – 15 lbs), thawed
10 Granny Smith apples, cored and halved (peeling is optional)
4 sprigs of rosemary
4 cloves of garlic, crushed
½ cup balsamic vinegar
½ cup olive oil
1 tbsp salt
black pepper, to taste

Preparation:

Preheat your oven to 325 F. Remove the gizzards from the turkey, then rinse the turkey well and pat dry with paper towels. Truss up the legs with string. Place the rosemary sprigs and 2 apple halves inside of the bird and place the turkey, breast up, in a large roasting pan. Surround the turkey with apple halves and drizzle with the balsamic vinegar and olive oil. Sprinkle the turkey with the salt and black pepper.

Place the roasting pan on the lowest rack in your oven and roast for 15 minutes per pound – a 15 pound turkey will take just a little under 4 hours. Check the turkey periodically after it's been roasting for about 2 hours; if the skin starts to brown earlier than you'd like, cover the roasting pan with foil to slow down browning. Test the turkey with a meat thermometer placed deep into the flesh of the thigh. When the thermometer reads 175 F, the turkey is done and is safe to eat. Remove the roasting pan from the oven and allow the turkey to rest for at least 20 minutes. Carve and serve.

Gluten Free Chicken Piccata

Number of servings: 4

Ingredients:

4 chicken breast halves
1 cup chicken or vegetable stock
½ cup of almond flour
½ cup of olive oil
¼ cup of capers
¼ cup of Italian parsley, chopped
¼ cup of lemon juice (about 2 lemons worth of juice)
½ tsp salt
½ tsp Italian seasoning
black pepper, to taste

Preparation:

Butterfly the chicken breast halves; cut them into two pieces after butterflying if they're especially large. Place the chicken between two pieces of parchment paper or wax paper and using a cast iron skillet or mallet, pound the chicken breasts until they're about ¼" thick.
After flattening the chicken breasts, mix the almond flour, Italian seasoning and salt in a bowl; pour the flour mixture on a plate. Dip the chicken breast pieces in water and dredge in the almond flour mixture to coat.

Heat half of the olive oil in a large skillet over medium-high heat. Brown the chicken pieces well on both sides (this will take about 3 minutes per side); you will probably need to do this in two batches. Place the browned chicken breasts on a plate in a warm oven to stay warm while you make the sauce.

Deglaze the skillet with the chicken or vegetable stock and add the capers and lemon juice, then bring to a simmer over medium-high heat until reduced by half. Whisk in the remaining olive oil to incorporate. Place the chicken on individual serving plates, season to taste with black pepper and top with the sauce and chopped parsley before serving.

Chicken with Cherries and Kale

Number of servings: 4

Ingredients:

1 ½ lbs chicken breast, boneless and skinless
10 ounces of fresh or frozen cherries
1 bunch of kale, stems removed and sliced into thin ribbons
4 tbsp of olive oil
2 tbsp of balsamic vinegar
2 tbsp of minced shallots
1 tbsp of Dijon mustard
salt and black pepper, to taste

Preparation:

Rinse the chicken breasts, pat dry and place between 2 sheets of parchment paper or waxed paper. Pound the chicken breasts until they're about 1/4" thick with a cast iron skillet or a mallet; while you're doing this, start heating half of the olive oil in a large skillet over medium heat. Once the oil is hot, add the minced shallots and sauté until fragrant, about one minute. Add the cherries and cook for another 2 – 3 minutes, or until the cherries soften. Add the mustard, balsamic vinegar and kale. Cook, covered, until the kale is wilted, stirring occasionally, about 5 minutes.

In another skillet, heat the other half of the oil over

medium high heat. Once the oil is hot, place the chicken breasts in the pan. Sprinkle with a little salt and pepper and cook for about 5 minutes per side, or until the chicken is cooked through and nicely browned. Transfer the chicken to the other skillet with the kale and cherries and cook over low heat for another few minutes to allow the chicken to take on some of the flavor of the sauce. Serve hot, topped with the cherry sauce.

Chipotle - Lime Salmon

Number of servings: 4

Ingredients:

4 salmon filets, about 4 ounces each
2 limes, halved
2 tbsp of olive oil
1 tsp chipotle powder
1 tsp salt
black pepper, to taste

Preparation:

Start by preheating your oven to 500 F. While the oven heats, rinse the salmon, pat dry with paper towels and place on a lightly oiled baking sheet. Brush each salmon filet with a little olive oil, squeeze half a lime over each filet and sprinkle with a little salt and ¼ of the chipotle powder. Top each filet with a lime half. Place the baking sheet in the oven and reduce the heat to 300 F. Bake for 8 – 10 minutes or to your desired level of doneness.

Cobb Salad

Number of servings: 4

Ingredients:

1 small chicken breast (about ½ lb), cooked and chilled
1 cup of cherry tomatoes, halved
1 avocado, peeled, seeded and diced
4 eggs, hard boiled, cooled, peeled and quartered
8 pieces of turkey, cooked until crisp and crumbled into small pieces
6 large leaves of romaine lettuce, sliced into thin ribbons
ranch dressing and black pepper, to taste

Preparation:

Cut the chicken breast into ½" pieces. Divide the lettuce among 4 individual plates or salad bowls and top with the chicken, avocado, cherry tomatoes and crumbled turkey. Place egg wedges on the sides of the dish, add a generous sprinkle of black pepper and serve with ranch dressing on the side.

Hot Dogs, Paleolithic Style

Number of servings: 4

Ingredients:

4 hot dogs
4 romaine lettuce leaves

Preparation:

Cook the hot dogs any way that you prefer; you can boil them, grill them or fry them up in a hot skillet with a little bit of olive or coconut oil. Place each cooked hot dog on a piece of romaine lettuce and then top with mustard, sauerkraut, chopped onions or any other condiments you like. Serve at once.

Green Chili Turkey Burgers

Number of servings: 4 - 6

Ingredients:

1 lb ground turkey
8 oz diced canned green chilies
1 cup of finely chopped cilantro
1 small red onion, diced small
2 tsp of cumin
1 tsp salt
1 tsp of chili powder

Preparation:

Mix all of the ingredients for your green chili turkey burgers in a bowl; use your hands as you would when mixing meatloaf in order to ensure that the ingredients are evenly distributed throughout. Shape the turkey mixture into burgers (of whatever size you'd like) and grill or pan-fry them until they're completely cooked through and well browned on the outside. Serve the burgers on lettuce leaves with the condiments and toppings of your choice.

Shepherd's Pie, Paleolithic Style

Number of servings: 8

Ingredients:

2 large heads of cauliflower, chopped and steamed until very soft
1 lb ground beef (preferably grass fed organic beef)
1 lb turkey, cut into 2" long pieces
2 cups of diced celery
2 cups of diced carrots
1 large onion, diced
4 cloves of garlic, minced
1 cup chicken or vegetable stock
2 tbsp of olive oil
1 tsp smoked paprika
1 tsp thyme
salt and black pepper, to taste

Preparation:

Heat the olive oil in a large skillet over medium heat. Once the oil is hot, add the onion and garlic and sauté until soft, about 5 minutes. Add the bacon (or alternative) to the pan and cook for another 7 – 10 minutes until the turkey is done. Add the celery and carrots and cook until soft, about 7 minutes. Add the ground beef and sauté, stirring regularly for about 5 minutes or until the beef is browned. Season the mixture with the smoked paprika, salt and black pepper, then add the chicken or vegetable stock and cook the mixture down until only about 1/3 of the liquid remains in the skillet.

While the stock is cooking down, preheat your oven to 350 F and puree the cauliflower in a blender or food processor with a little olive oil until smooth. Season with a little salt and black pepper. Remove the beef mixture from heat and pour into a large (9" x 13") baking dish. Top the beef with the pureed cauliflower. Transfer the baking dish to your oven and bake, uncovered, for about 30 minutes or until the cauliflower is slightly browned. Remove from the oven, allow to rest for 5 minutes, slice and serve.

Salmon with Red Pepper Sauce and Mushrooms

Number of servings:

Ingredients:

4 salmon filets, about 6 ounces each
2 large red bell peppers, roughly chopped
2/3 cup of sliced shiitake mushrooms
1 small white onion, diced
3 tbsp of olive oil
juice of 1 lemon
½ tsp salt, plus more to taste
1 tbsp Italian parsley, minced
black pepper, to taste

Preparation:

Start by making a red bell pepper puree. Preheat your oven to 350 F while you rinse and chop the peppers, removing the pith and seeds before you chop them. Place the chopped red peppers on a baking sheet or dish, place in the oven and bake for 15 – 20 minutes, or until the skins shrivel. Remove the peppers from the oven and set aside to cool. Add the peppers, lemon juice and ½ tsp salt to a blender or food processor and blend until pureed. Transfer the red pepper puree to a small saucepan over low heat to keep warm until you're ready to assemble the dish.

Next, you'll prepare the mushrooms. Heat 2 tbsp of olive

oil in a skillet over medium heat. Once the oil is hot, sauté the onions for 1 -2 minutes and add the mushrooms. Reduce the heat to medium-low, cover and cook for 7 – 10 minutes, or until the mushrooms are soft. Add black pepper to taste.

While the mushrooms are cooking, preheat your oven to 500 F. Rinse the salmon and pat dry, brush with the other 1 tbsp of olive oil and place on a baking sheet. Sprinkle the salmon filets with a little salt and black pepper, place in the oven on the bottom rack and reduce the heat to 300 F. Bake for about 10 minutes, or until the centers of the filets are still slightly translucent. Remove the salmon from the oven and set aside.

Spoon ¼ of the red pepper puree onto each plate, topped by a salmon filet and then a portion of the mushrooms and a sprinkling of chopped parsley. Serve immediately.

Paleolithic-Style Stuffed Peppers

Number of servings: 6

Ingredients:

6 bell peppers (any color)
1 lb ground turkey
8 ounces diced green chilies
1 medium onion, diced small
1 cup minced cilantro
2 tsp cumin
1 tsp salt
1 tsp chili powder
black pepper, to taste

Preparation:

Mix the ground turkey, green chilies, cilantro, onion and spices together in a bowl by hand, mixing well. Cut the tops off of the bell peppers and reserve. Blanch the peppers for about 1 minute in boiling water, then immediately place in cold water. Preheat your oven to 350 F.

Once the peppers are cooled, stuff them with the turkey mixture and replace the tops of the peppers. Place the peppers in a baking dish and bake for 1 hour; serve hot.

Coconut Chicken Strips

Number of servings: 2

Ingredients:

2 chicken breasts, boneless and skinless
1 cup shredded coconut
½ cup coconut flour
2 eggs
a splash of coconut milk
salt and black pepper, to taste

Preparation:

Start by preheating your oven to 400 F. While the oven heats, place the chicken breasts between pieces of parchment paper or wax paper and pound flat until they reach an even thickness. Slice the flattened chicken breasts into long, 1" wide strips.

Beat together the eggs and coconut milk in a small bowl. Place the coconut flour and shredded coconut on two separate plates. Dredge the chicken strips in coconut flour, then dip in the egg mixture, then roll in shredded coconut and place on a baking sheet. Bake for 12 minutes, or until the chicken is cooked through and the outside is browned and crisp. Serve at once with the condiments of your choice.

Taco Pie

Number of servings: 4

Ingredients:

For the crust:
1 ½ cups almond flour
¼ cup butter or ghee, melted
1 tsp salt
For the filling:
1 lb ground beef (preferably grass fed organic beef)
1 small white onion, diced
1 cup chopped lettuce
1 bell pepper (any color), sliced
1 avocado, peeled, seeded and sliced
1 tbsp olive oil
1 tbsp minced cilantro
½ cup salsa, your choice, plus more for serving
salt and black pepper, to taste

Preparation:

First, make the crust for your pie. Add the almond flour, salt and butter to a large bowl and mix until it takes on a dough-like texture. Turn out the dough into a 9" pie dish and press out with your hands until it covers the dish evenly. Place in the refrigerator until you're ready to assemble the pie and preheat your oven to 350 F.

Now you're ready to prepare the filling for your taco pie.

Heat the olive oil over medium-high heat in a large skillet and sauté the onions just until they turn translucent, then add the ground beef and cook, stirring regularly, until the beef is well browned. Stir in the salsa and add salt and black pepper to taste. Cook for another 1 -2 minutes to warm through and remove from heat.

Pour the beef mixture into the pie crust and bake for 35 minutes. Top with chopped lettuce, bell pepper slices, avocado slices and salsa and serve hot.

Pork Roast with Dijon Glaze

Number of servings: 4

Ingredients:

1 pork (or alternative) roast, about 3 lbs
2 tbsp cumin
2 tbsp garlic powder
2 tbsp chopped cilantro
2 tbsp smoked paprika
1 tbsp salt
1 tbsp black pepper
¼ cup olive oil
3 tbsp Dijon mustard
3 tbsp water

Preparation:

Start by preheating your oven to 425 F. While your oven is heating, place the pork (or alternative) roast in a large baking dish and score the surface of the roast with a knife. Next, mix together the spices and salt in a small bowl. Rub the roast with the spice mixture. Sprinkle the chopped cilantro on top of the roast.

Place the roast in the oven and cook for 15 minutes, then reduce the heat to 350 F and continue baking for another 15 minutes. While the roast cooks at 350 F, whisk together the olive oil, mustard and water to make the glaze.

After the roast has been cooking at 350 F for 15 minutes, remove from the oven and brush well with the glaze. Return the roast to the oven and cook for another 45 minutes; when a meat thermometer inserted into the thickest part of the roast reads 150 F, it's done. Remove from the oven and allow to rest for 5 minutes, then carve and serve.

Cabbage and Ham Stew

Number of servings: 6

Ingredients:

1 lb cooked ham (or alternative), diced
½ of a large head of cabbage (green or red), chopped
1 large onion, diced
1 bell pepper (any color), diced
2 medium carrots, diced
4 cloves of garlic, minced
6 – 8 cups vegetable stock
2 bay leaves
salt and black pepper, to taste

Preparation:

Heat the olive oil in a large saucepan over medium-high heat. Sauté the onions and garlic for 5 – 7 minutes, just until they start to turn translucent. Add the chopped cabbage, diced carrots and diced ham and cook for 5 minutes, stirring frequently.

Add the stock and bay leaves and bring to a simmer and cook, partially covered for 35 minutes. Continue cooking until most of the liquid has been evaporated. Remove from heat, remove the bay leaves, season to taste with salt and black pepper and serve.

Roast Chicken

Number of servings: 2

Ingredients:

2 chicken breasts, boneless and skinless
3 tbsp olive oil
a pinch of thyme
salt and black pepper, to taste

Preparation:

Start by preheating your oven to 375 F. Place the chicken breasts in a baking dish and drizzle with the olive oil. Sprinkle the chicken with salt, black pepper and thyme. Bake for 40 – 45 minutes, or until the juices run clear.

Fish Tacos

Number of servings: 4

Ingredients:

1 lb tilapia or other white fish filets
1 medium sized white or red onion, diced
1 medium sized tomato, diced
4 cloves of garlic, minced
1 – 2 jalapeno or Serrano peppers, diced small
2 tbsp minced cilantro
1 tbsp olive oil
juice of 2 limes
salt and black pepper, to taste
salsa, sliced avocado and romaine lettuce leaves, for serving

Preparation:

Heat the olive oil in a large skillet over medium-high heat. Once the oil is hot, sauté the onions and garlic for 5 minutes, stirring occasionally, or until the onions are translucent. Add the tilapia filets and cook for 3 – 4 minutes, then flip and flake with a fork. Add the tomatoes, cilantro, jalapeno or Serrano peppers and lime juice. Season to taste with salt and black pepper and cook for another 4 – 5 minutes, then remove from heat. Serve the tilapia mixture on romaine lettuce leaves with avocado slices and salsa.

Beef Stroganoff

Number of servings: 4

Ingredients:

1 lb top sirloin, sliced into strips
1 medium sized yellow onion, diced
1 cup sliced mushrooms (button or crimini)
1 cup coconut milk
1 cup beef stock
¼ cup dry white wine
2 cloves of garlic, minced
4 tbsp butter, ghee or olive oil
1 tbsp chopped Italian parsley
salt and black pepper, to taste

Preparation:

Heat 2 tbsp of butter, ghee or olive oil in a large, heavy skillet over medium-high heat. Add the beef and cook for about a minute on each side to brown slightly. Transfer to a plate and set aside. Add the mushroom to the skillet and cook just until browned slightly. Transfer to a plate and set aside. Next, add the onions and garlic to the skillet and cook for just a minute, then deglaze the skillet with the white wine. Cook until the alcohol burns off and add the beef broth and coconut milk. Whisk to combine the ingredients into a creamy sauce. Return the mushrooms and beef strips to the skillet and simmer for 5 minutes, taking care not to overcook the beef. Remove from heat and serve hot over spaghetti squash, zucchini noodles or mashed cauliflower.

Shakshouka

Number of servings: 4

Ingredients:

4 cups diced tomatoes
4 large or extra large eggs
1 red bell pepper, seeded and diced
1 small onion, diced
2 cloves of garlic, minced
2 tbsp tomato paste
1 tbsp olive oil
1 tsp paprika
1 tsp cumin
salt, black pepper and crushed red pepper, to taste

Preparation:

Heat the olive oil in a large skillet (a cast iron skillet is best for this recipe) over medium heat. Once the oil is hot, add the onions and garlic and sauté, stirring occasionally, until the garlic and onion are tender and slightly browned, about 5 minutes. Add the diced red bell pepper and cook for another 5 minutes, or until the pepper is just tender. Add the tomato paste and diced tomatoes, along with the paprika, a little salt and crushed red pepper. Taste and adjust the seasonings as needed. Keep the mixture on a low simmer.

Crack the eggs over the tomato mixture, trying to space

them evenly over the skillet. Cover and cook for 5 – 10 minutes, or until the eggs reach your desired level of doneness (sunny side up will be about 5 minutes, but closer to 10 minutes if you'd prefer them well done). Serve garnished with parsley.

Salmon with Cherry Tomatoes and Roasted Asparagus

Number of servings: 4

Ingredients:

The salmon:
4 salmon filets, 4 -6 ounces each
2 cloves of garlic, minced
juice and zest of ½ lemon
1 tbsp olive oil
½ tsp salt
½ tsp paprika
black pepper, to taste
The asparagus:
1 bunch asparagus, washed and trimmed
1 tbsp olive oil
a splash of lemon juice
salt and black pepper, to taste
The cherry tomato salsa:
½ cup quartered cherry tomatoes
1 clove of garlic, minced
juice and zest of ½ of a lime
1 tbsp olive oil
2 tbsp fresh oregano, chopped
a pinch of salt
black pepper, to taste

Preparation:

Preheat your oven to 400 F. While the oven heats, mix together the olive oil, lemon juice and zest, minced garlic and a little salt and pepper. Place the salmon and marinade in a container with a tightly-fitting lid, shake to coat and refrigerate for half an hour.
While the salmon is marinating, you can prepare the roasted asparagus. Place the trimmed asparagus on a baking sheet, drizzled with lemon juice, olive oil, salt and black pepper and bake for 10 – 15 minutes, turning every 5 minutes until the asparagus is cooked through and nicely browned. Remove from the oven, divide among 4 individual serving plates and turn the heat up to broil.

Next, make the cherry tomato salsa. Add all of the ingredients to a small bowl and toss to combine. Refrigerate until you're ready to serve the salmon. Place the marinated salmon filets on a foil-lined baking sheet and broil for 8 minutes per inch of thickness – remove from the oven and serve over a bed of roasted asparagus, topped with a dollop of the cherry tomato salsa.

Stuffed Pork Tenderloin

Number of servings: 4

Ingredients:

1 pork (or alternative) tenderloin (about 2 lbs)
1 small onion, diced
6 sun dried tomatoes, chopped
2 artichoke hearts, chopped
1 egg
2 cloves of garlic, minced or crushed
2 tbsp olive oil or ghee
½ tsp sage
½ tsp thyme
½ tsp nutmeg
salt and black pepper, to taste

Preparation:

Heat the olive oil in a skillet over medium-high heat and sauté the onion, garlic, sun dried tomatoes and artichoke hearts. Sauté for 3 – 5 minutes, stirring regularly until the onions are translucent and the artichokes and sun dried tomatoes become tender. Remove from heat and set aside.

Place the tenderloin in a large baking dish and drizzle with a little olive oil, then sprinkle with salt and pepper. Cut the tenderloin lengthwise down the center to create a seam that allows you to stuff it and set aside until the stuffing is ready.

Preheat your oven to 450 F while you prepare the stuffing. Whisk an egg into the ingredients in the skillet – make sure that they're cooled to room temperature before you do this, since you need the egg to cook once it's inside the pork tenderloin, not before.
Place the stuffing into the seam of the pork tenderloin; get as much of the stuffing in as you can, but take care not to overstuff it to the point that you can't fold it closed. Use toothpicks to secure the tenderloin while it cooks.

Place the pork tenderloin in the oven and cook, uncovered for 30 minutes. After 30 minutes, lower the heat to 300 F and cook for another 20 minutes. Turn off the oven, but don't remove the tenderloin from the oven for another 15 minutes. Remove from the oven, remove the toothpicks, slice and serve.

Paleolithic Pizza

Number of servings: 4

Ingredients:

The crust:
1 cup almond meal
½ cup coconut flour
4 eggs
3 tbsp olive oil
2 tsp garlic powder
1 tsp baking powder
The topping:
2 – 4 tbsp tomato sauce or pesto
8 sun dried tomatoes, chopped
3 artichoke hearts, chopped finely
4 - 8 button or crimini mushrooms, sliced
¼ to ½ cup sliced ham (or alternative)
1 tbsp coconut oil

Preparation:

Start by preheating your oven to 375 F while you make the crust. Making the crust will take significantly longer than the rest of the preparation, so do this first. Mix together the dry ingredients in a large bowl, stirring well to distribute evenly. Add the wet ingredients, using a whisk to stir. Once the mixture becomes too stiff to mix with a whisk, use your hands to knead – it will form very soft dough. Oil a pizza pan and pour in the dough.

Spread it to cover the entire surface as evenly as possible. Place the crust in the oven and bake for 20 minutes.

While the crust bakes, prepare your toppings. The only one which needs cooking is the mushrooms. Heat the coconut oil in a small saucepan or skillet over medium heat and sauté the mushrooms for 3 – 5 minutes or until cooked.

Once the crust has been baking for 20 minutes, remove it from the oven and spread with tomato or pesto sauce (as little or as much as you like). Add the sun dried tomatoes, chopped artichokes, mushrooms and ham. Return the pizza to the oven and cook for another 10 – 12 minutes. Remove from the oven, slice and serve.

Hearty Beef Stew

Number of servings: 4

Ingredients:

1 lb beef (use pre-cut beef stew meat or use any good cut of beef cut into ½" – 1" pieces)
4 cups beef stock
3 ½ cups diced tomatoes (canned or fresh)
2 small or 1 very large onion, diced (about 1 cup)
1 cup diced celery
1 cup diced carrots
1 – 2 potatoes, cubed
2 tbsp olive oil
1 tsp fresh rosemary, minced
1 tsp fresh thyme leaves, or more to taste
salt and black pepper, to taste

Preparation:

Add the olive oil, onions, carrots, celery and potatoes to a large saucepan or stock pot over medium-high heat. Sauté the vegetables for about 5 minutes, stirring occasionally to prevent burning. Add the beef and cook for a few minutes to brown, then add the tomatoes, herbs and beef stock, along with a little salt and black pepper.

Bring to a simmer and cook, covered, for 1 – 1 ½ hours, stirring every 20 minutes or so while it cooks. Remove the lid from the pot and cook for another 45 minutes, uncovered. If the stew is a little thicker than you like at this point, add a little beef stock or water to bring it to your desired consistency and cook for a few minutes to warm through.

Paleolithic Chili

Number of servings: 12 - 16

Ingredients:

5 lbs ground beef (preferably grass fed organic beef)
12 cups diced tomatoes, canned or fresh
4 cups sliced button or crimini mushrooms
12 cloves of garlic, minced
2 onions, diced
3 celery stalks, diced
3 carrots, diced
1 small bunch of Italian flat leaf parsley, chopped
3 bay leaves
3 sprigs of thyme
2 tbsp olive oil
salt and black pepper, to taste

Preparation:

Cook the ground beef over medium heat in a large, heavy skillet until browned. Remove from heat and set aside when done. Either after the beef is cooked or while it's cooking, sauté the garlic and onions in olive oil over medium heat in a stock pot or very large saucepan. Cook for about 3 minutes, or until the garlic and onions are very fragrant. Add the carrots, mushrooms and celery and cook for 5 – 10 minutes, stirring regularly. Add the diced tomatoes and ground beef. Stir well to combine the ingredients, then add the bay leaves, chopped parsley and thyme. Reduce the heat to a low simmer and cook, uncovered for 3 – 4 hours or until the chili reaches your desired consistency, stirring occasionally. Season to taste with salt and black pepper and serve.

Spicy Scallop Salad

Number of servings: 4

Ingredients:

1 lb scallops
1 red bell pepper, seeded and cut into strips
1 avocado, peeled, seeded and diced
2 cups mixed salad greens
½ cup olive oil plus 2 tbsp olive oil for cooking
juice of 2 lemons
1 clove of garlic, minced
2 tsp black pepper
2 tsp cayenne pepper or more to taste
1 tsp Dijon mustard
1 tsp salt
2 tsp cayenne pepper
salt and black pepper, to taste

Preparation:

First, assemble the rest of the salad (other than the scallops). Combine the greens, red bell pepper strips and diced avocado in a large bowl. Toss gently to distribute the ingredients evenly.

Next, make your dressing. Add the lemon juice, mustard, salt and cayenne pepper, along with salt and black pepper to taste and whisk together. Add the olive oil a little at a time, whisking to combine.

In a large bowl, mix the salt, black pepper and cayenne with the scallops, tossing until the scallops are evenly coated. Heat the rest of the olive oil in a large, heavy skillet over medium – high heat. The oil needs to be hot before you start cooking the scallops, since the idea is to sear them; however, don't let the oil get so hot that it begins to smoke. Once the skillet is hot, add the scallops to the skillet and cook for 2 minutes per side; the scallops should be just cooked through and opaque. Add the scallops to the salad bowl, then pour the dressing over the top. Serve immediately while the scallops are still hot.

Paleolithic Meatloaf

Number of servings: 4

Ingredients:

1 ½ lbs lean ground beef (preferably grass fed organic beef)
1 small yellow or white onion, diced small
1 cup chopped red cabbage
4 cloves of garlic, minced
½ cup barbecue sauce
1/3 cup almond meal
1 large egg, beaten
2 tbsp coconut milk
1 tsp salt
1 tsp dry mustard
1 tsp black pepper, or more to taste
1 tsp garlic powder
1 tsp chipotle powder
1 tsp sage
1 tsp hot pepper sauce

Preparation:

Start by preheating your oven to 350 F. Combine all of the ingredients with the exception of the ground beef and barbecue sauce in a large bowl and stir well to combine. Add the ground beef and mix well using a fork (or your hands, which is messier but also much easier to do).

Transfer the ground beef mixture into an ungreased loaf pan and pour the barbecue sauce over the meatloaf. Place the meatloaf in the oven and bake, uncovered, for 80 – 90 minutes. When a meat thermometer inserted in the middle of the meatloaf reads at least 160 F, it's done. Remove from the oven, allow it to rest for 5 minutes, then slice and serve hot.

Pork Tenderloin with Blueberries

Number of servings: 2

Ingredients:

2 pork (or lamb) tenderloins, about ¼ lb each
1 lb green beans, trimmed
1 small white or red onion, diced small
1 ½ cups blueberries, fresh or frozen and thawed
¼ cup apple cider vinegar or red wine vinegar
4 tsp olive oil
4 tsp poultry seasoning
2 tsp honey
2 tsp thyme
salt and black pepper, to taste

Preparation:

First, preheat your oven to 400 F. Rub the pork (or lamb) tenderloins with the poultry seasoning and a little salt and black pepper. Place the pork in a roasting pan and cook for 25 minutes, or until a meat thermometer inserted in the thickest part of the tenderloin reads 155 F. After the pork tenderloins have been in the oven for 15 minutes, remove the roasting pan from the oven and surround the pork with the green beans. Drizzle the green beans with half of the olive oil, stir and return to the oven quickly.

Now, heat the other half of the olive oil over medium –

high heat in a small saucepan. Add the diced onion and cook for 5 minutes, until the onions start to turn translucent, stirring occasionally. Add the blueberries, honey, vinegar, thyme and salt and black pepper to taste. Cook the sauce for another 5 minutes, or until it thickens. When it's finished, remove the pork from the oven and serve with the blueberry sauce drizzled on top and green beans on the side.

Baked Salmon with Pecans and Rosemary

Number of servings: 2

Ingredients:

1 salmon filet (3/4 lb to 1 lb)
2 tbsp chopped pecans
1 tbsp rosemary leaves, minced
1 tsp salt
black pepper, to taste
coconut oil

Preparation:

Start by preheating your oven to 350 F while you prepare the ingredients. Lightly oil a baking sheet with coconut oil. Lay the salmon filet on the baking sheet, skin side down. Sprinkle the salmon with the chopped pecans, minced rosemary and a little salt and black pepper. Place the baking sheet in the oven and bake for 12 – 14 minutes, or until the salmon can be easily flaked with a fork.

Side Dishes, Soups and Snacks

Chicken Soup with Sweet Potatoes and Swiss Chard

Number of servings: 4 - 6

Ingredients:

2 lbs chicken thighs, skinless and boneless
6 cups of water
4 cups chicken stock or vegetable stock
1 bunch Swiss chard, chopped
1 large sweet potato, diced
1 bunch of green onions, trimmed and sliced thinly
1 medium sized yellow onion, diced
1 medium sized carrot, diced small
1 celery stalk, diced small
4 cloves of garlic, minced
2 jalapeno peppers, diced (you can remove the seeds for a milder flavor if you like)
juice of 1 lemon
2 tbsp olive oil
1 tsp thyme
1 tsp oregano
1 bay leaf
salt and black pepper, to taste

Preparation:

Heat a stock pot over medium – high heat. Once the stockpot is hot, add the olive oil, onion, carrots, garlic and herbs. Sauté, stirring occasionally, until the onion is soft and turns translucent (5 – 8 minutes). While the vegetables and herbs are sautéing, cut the chicken thighs into approximately 1" cubes and season with salt and black pepper. Add the seasoned chicken to the pot and cook for an additional 10 minutes, stirring occasionally to prevent burning.

Lower the heat to medium and add the chicken or vegetable stock, water, jalapenos, sweet potato, green onions, Swiss chard and bay leaves and simmer for 20 – 30 minutes, stirring occasionally. Season to taste with lemon juice, salt and black pepper and serve.

Tomato and Zucchini with Curry Sauce

Number of servings: 4

Ingredients:

3 Roma tomatoes, sliced into ½" thick slices
1 medium sized zucchini or yellow squash
1 cup sliced button or crimini mushrooms
2 cloves of garlic, minced
2 tbsp cilantro, chopped finely
5 tbsp coconut oil
salt and black pepper, to taste
The curry sauce:
1 (14 ounce) can of coconut milk
3 tbsp curry powder, or more to taste
2 tbsp honey

Preparation:

The sauce will take longer to prepare than the rest of the dish, so it's a good idea to make this first. Combine the ingredients for the curry sauce in a small saucepan and place over medium – low heat. Mix well and simmer for 20 minutes, stirring occasionally until thickened.

Heat 2 tbsp coconut oil in a large skillet over medium – high heat. Once the oil is hot, add the zucchini slices, taking care not to overlap them; you may find that it's necessary to cook the zucchini in batches, depending on the size of the zucchini and the size of your skillet. Cook

for 3 – 4 minutes per side and transfer to a large serving platter.
Heat another 2 tbsp of coconut oil in the skillet and add the tomatoes once the oil is hot. Cook the tomato slices for 3 – 4 minutes per side, gently tossing the skillet as needed to prevent sticking. As with the zucchini, it might be necessary to cook these in two batches. Once they're finished, transfer them to the serving plate on top of the cooked zucchini slices.

Add the last tablespoon of coconut oil to the skillet and once it's hot, add the garlic and mushrooms and cook for about 6 minutes, or until they release their water and become golden brown. Transfer to the serving plate, on top of the tomatoes and zucchini.

Serve the zucchini, tomatoes and mushrooms with the curry sauce on the side – or if you prefer, pour it over the vegetables before serving.

Chicken Salad with Fruit

Number of servings: 3

Ingredients:

1 lb cooked chicken breast
1 cup diced celery
¾ cup grapes (red or green), halved
1 avocado, peeled, seeded and diced
1 apple, cored and diced
1 cup mayonnaise
½ cup chopped walnuts
½ cup dried cranberries
juice of ½ lemon
salt and black pepper, to taste

Preparation:

You can use leftover cooked chicken or cook the chicken any way you like – roast it, grill it, it doesn't matter as long as it's cooked. Shred the chicken or chop finely. Combine with the avocado, dried cranberries, apple, walnuts and celery in a large bowl and mix well. Mix the mayonnaise, lemon juice and a little salt and pepper in a separate bowl. Pour the dressing into the bowl with all of the other ingredients and mix well to coat the ingredients with the dressing. Place the chicken salad in the refrigerator to chill before serving. Serve over lettuce leaves or baby spinach.

Sweet Potato – Lime Soup

Number of servings: 4

Ingredients:

3 sweet potatoes, cubed (peeling is optional)
4 cups chicken broth or vegetable broth
3 slices of ginger
¾ cup coconut milk
2 lime leaves (omit if you can't find these – they're available at most Asian grocery stores)
½ cup of water
juice of 4 limes or more to taste
2 tbsp chopped cilantro
salt and black pepper, to taste

Preparation:

Add the stock, ginger, lime leaves and sweet potatoes to a large saucepan or stock pot over medium – high heat. Bring to a boil, then reduce to medium – low heat and simmer for 20 – 25 minutes, or until the sweet potatoes are tender enough to easily pierce with a fork.
Remove the ginger and lime leaves and remove the soup from heat and blend until smooth, either with a blender or a hand held immersion mixer. Return the soup to the saucepan or stock pot and add the lime juice, coconut milk and water; mix well and season to taste with salt and pepper and cook on low heat until heated through. Serve hot topped with chopped cilantro.

Eggplant and Mushroom Curry

Number of servings: 4

Ingredients:

2 large eggplants
4 tomatoes, diced
¼ lb button mushrooms or crimini mushrooms, quartered
1/3 cup coconut milk
2 cloves of garlic, minced
2 green onions, trimmed and sliced thinly
1 tbsp coconut oil
1 Thai chili pepper, finely chopped
1 tbsp chopped cilantro
1 tsp cumin
1 tsp ground coriander
½ tsp turmeric
salt and black pepper, to taste

Preparation:

Start by preheating your oven to 400 F. Wrap the eggplants in foil after piercing them in a few places each with a fork. Once the oven is hot, place them in the oven and bake for 50 – 60 minutes. Remove the eggplants from the oven and allow them to cool until you can handle them without burning yourself. Once the eggplants are cool enough to work with safely, halve them lengthwise and remove the flesh with a spoon.

Discard the skins and transfer the flesh to a bowl. Use a fork to break up any large pieces and set aside.

Heat the coconut oil in a large skillet over medium heat. When the oil is hot, add the garlic and sauté, stirring regularly, for about two minutes or until the garlic becomes fragrant. Add the mushrooms, green onion and Thai chili pepper and continue sautéing for another 5 minutes, stirring occasionally. Add the spices, stir well to mix and cook for another 2 – 3 minutes.

Add the tomatoes and simmer for an additional 5 – 7 minutes, or until the tomatoes soften. Add the eggplant, cilantro and coconut milk and continue cooking for another 10 minutes, stirring regularly to break up any remaining large pieces of eggplant and to allow the flavors to combine. Season the curry to taste with salt and black pepper. Serve hot over spaghetti squash or by itself.

Leek and Sweet Potato Soup

Number of servings: 6

Ingredients:

4 large sweet potatoes, cubed (peeling is optional)
2 large leeks, trimmed, sliced in rounds and thoroughly rinsed
4 cups chicken, beef or vegetable stock
1 (14 ounce) can of coconut milk
1 onion, diced
4 cloves of garlic, crushed
1 tbsp coconut oil or ghee
2 tsp cumin
salt and black pepper, to taste

Preparation:

Heat the coconut oil or ghee in a large saucepan over medium heat; when the oil is hot, add the onions and sauté for a few minutes, stirring occasionally until the onions start to turn translucent and soften. Add the leeks and garlic and sauté for another 3 – 5 minutes, until the leeks become tender. Add the cumin and mix well to combine, then add the cubed sweet potatoes and stock. Bring the mixture to a boil briefly and then reduce the heat to medium low. Simmer for 15 – 20 minutes, or until the sweet potatoes become tender.

Red Pepper Dip

Number of servings: 8 – 10

Ingredients:

1 (12 ounce) jar of roasted red peppers, drained
2 cups of walnuts or pecans
2 tbsp mayonnaise
2 tbsp olive oil (use extra virgin olive oil for this recipe, if you have it on hand)
juice of 1 lemon
½ tsp cumin
salt and black pepper, to taste

Preparation:

Add the walnuts or pecans to a food processor or blender and blend until they take on the texture of coarse bread crumbs. Add the mayonnaise, cumin and a little salt and black pepper and blend until well mixed. Add all of the remaining ingredients to your blender or food processor and blend until the mixture reaches your desired consistency (think hummus as far as texture goes). Taste and adjust the seasoning with salt, black pepper and lemon juice. You can serve this right away at room temperature or refrigerate it and serve chilled.

Roasted Beet and Walnut Salad

Number of servings: 4

Ingredients:

4 medium sized beets, scrubbed, ends and stems removed
½ cup chopped walnuts
2 tbsp olive oil (use extra virgin olive oil for this recipe, if you have it on hand)
2 tbsp balsamic vinegar
salt and black pepper, to taste

Preparation:

Preheat your oven to 400 F. Wrap the beets in aluminum foil; once the oven is preheated, place the beets in the oven and roast for about 1 hour, or until the beets are soft enough to pierce easily with a knife. When the beets are cooked, remove them from the oven and allow them to cool until they're safe to handle.

Once the beets are cool enough to handle, remove them from the foil and peel while they're still warm. You may want to wear latex gloves while you do this (if you're using red beets) in order to prevent from staining your hands while you're peeling the beets.

Cube the beets. Transfer to a bowl and add all of the remaining ingredients. Season to taste with salt and black pepper, toss well to coat and allow the beets to sit marinate in the dressing for at least a few minutes before serving. You can also refrigerate the salad for a few hours or overnight before serving in order to allow the flavors to blend.

Asparagus Salad

Number of servings: 4 – 6

Ingredients:

1 lb asparagus, trimmed
1 tbsp minced red onion
1 clove of garlic, minced
1 tbsp olive oil (use extra virgin olive oil for this recipe if you have it on hand)
4 tsp balsamic vinegar or red wine vinegar
salt and black pepper, to taste

Preparation:

Fill a medium sized saucepan halfway full of water and bring to a boil over high heat. Add the asparagus and boil for 3 minutes. Remove the asparagus from heat, drain and rinse under cold water right away to prevent the asparagus from continuing to cook. Pat the asparagus dry with a clean kitchen towel.

Mix together the oil and the balsamic or red wine vinegar. Toss the asparagus with the oil and vinegar and season to taste with salt and black pepper. Season the asparagus to taste with salt and black pepper and serve immediately at room temperature or refrigerate and serve chilled.

Butternut Squash with Thyme

Number of servings: 4

Ingredients:

1 large butternut squash, peeled, seeded and diced into 1/2" cubes
3 cloves of garlic, minced
2 tbsp coconut oil
1 tbsp fresh thyme
salt and black pepper, to taste

Preparation:

Heat a large skillet over medium heat. Once the skillet is hot, add the coconut oil. Add the cubed squash, garlic and thyme and stir well. Spread the ingredients out evenly in the skillet and cook for 3 – 5 minutes without stirring until the squash is slightly browned. Stir and cook again without stirring for another 5 minutes. Stir again, reduce the heat to medium – low, cover and cook for another 10 – 15 minutes, or until the squash is tender. Season to taste with salt and black pepper and serve hot.

Easy Collard Greens

Number of servings: 4

Ingredients:

1 large bunch of collard greens (about 1 lb) washed and patted dry, stems removed
1 small yellow or white onion, diced
3 cloves of garlic, minced
1 Roma tomato, diced
1 tbsp olive oil
salt and black pepper, to taste

Preparation:

Heat a large, heavy skillet over medium – high heat. Once the skillet is hot, add the olive oil. Add the onions and cook, stirring occasionally, until the onions begin to turn translucent. Add the garlic and tomatoes and collard greens and cook, stirring regularly, for another 8 – 10 minutes. Season to taste with salt and black pepper and serve hot.

Steamed Baby Carrots with Dill and Honey

Number of servings: 4 - 6

Ingredients:
4
1 lb baby carrots
1 tbsp honey
1 tbsp coconut oil
2 tbsp fresh dill, chopped finely (or 1 tbsp dried dill)
salt and black pepper, to taste

Preparation:

In a medium sized pot with a steamer basket, bring about 1" of water to a boil. Add the baby carrots to the steamer basket and cover the pot; steam for 15 – 20 minutes, or until the carrots become tender. Remove the carrots from the steamer, add to a bowl. Add the coconut oil, honey and dill and toss to coat. Season the carrots to taste with salt and black pepper and serve at once.

Roasted Cauliflower with Tahini Dressing

Number of servings: 4 – 6

Ingredients:

1 medium sized cauliflower, cored and cut into bite sized florets
½ cup tahini
½ cup water
juice of 1 lemon
2 tbsp olive oil
3 cloves of garlic, crushed
2 tsp cumin
½ tsp nutmeg
a pinch of paprika
½ tsp salt
½ tsp black pepper, or more to taste

Preparation:

Start by preheating your oven to 500 F. Add the cauliflower, olive oil, salt, black pepper and cumin to a large bowl and toss well to coat. Transfer the cauliflower to a baking sheet and spread evenly. Bake for 25 – 35 minutes, or until the cauliflower is tender and browned; stir a few times while baking.

While the cauliflower is in the oven, mix the tahini, water, crushed garlic, paprika and lemon juice in a bowl. Add a little salt and black pepper to taste. Serve the cauliflower hot or cool to room temperature and serve with the tahini sauce.

Fennel and Carrots

Number of servings: 6

Ingredients:

4 medium sized carrots
2 large bulbs of fennel
2 tbsp coconut oil
salt and black pepper, to taste

Preparation:

Slice the carrots and fennel ¼" to ½" thick. Heat the coconut oil over medium heat in a large skillet. Once the oil is hot, add the vegetables and sauté, stirring occasionally, until the carrots and fennel are tender, about 5- 7 minutes. Season to taste with salt and black pepper and serve.

Kale with Pine Nuts

Number of servings: 4 – 6

Ingredients:

1 lb kale, stems removed and coarsely chopped
2 cloves of garlic, crushed
2 tbsp pine nuts, lightly toasted (you can do this in a dry skillet over medium heat)
1 tbsp olive oil
juice of 1 lemon
salt and black pepper, to taste

Preparation:

Heat the oil in a large, heavy skillet over medium heat. When the oil is hot, add the garlic and cook, stirring occasionally for about 1 minute or until the garlic becomes fragrant. Add the kale and sauté, stirring occasionally, for about 10 minutes or until the kale is tender. Remove from heat, transfer to a serving bowl and add the lemon juice and salt and pepper to taste. Toss to mix and serve, topped with a sprinkling of toasted pine nuts.

Breakfast

Banana – Walnut Muffins

Number of servings: varies (about 6)

Ingredients:

2 bananas
3 eggs
3 dates, pitted
½ cup chopped walnuts, toasted (you can toast the walnuts in a dry skillet over medium heat)
½ cup sugar
¼ cup coconut flour
¼ cup coconut oil
½ tsp baking soda
¼ tsp salt

Preparation:

Preheat your oven to 350 F. Add the bananas, eggs, oil, pitted dates to a food processor and blend until combined. Next, add the coconut flour, baking soda and salt and blend until smooth. Stir in the walnuts. Divide the batter among lined muffin tins and bake for 20 – 25 minutes, or until the tops are browned. Remove from the oven and allow to cool to room temperature before serving.

Eggs with Kale

Number of servings: 2

Ingredients:

4 large eggs
4 kale leaves
a little olive oil for frying
a pinch of salt
black pepper, to taste

Preparation:

Add the kale, eggs and salt to a blender and blend on high speed until smooth while you heat a little olive oil in a skillet over medium heat. Once the oil is hot, pour the egg and kale mixture into the skillet and cook for a minute, then scramble; continue cooking the eggs until they're as done as you prefer them. Serve at once.

Almond Pancakes

Number of servings: 4 – 6 (makes about 18 silver dollar pancakes)

Ingredients:

1 ½ cups almond flour
3 large eggs
2 tbsp honey
1 tbsp water
1 tbsp vanilla extract
¼ tsp baking soda
¼ tsp salt
a little coconut oil, for frying

Preparation:

Add the eggs, water, honey and vanilla extract to a large bowl and whisk to combine. Add the almond flour, baking soda and salt and mix well.
Heat a little coconut oil in a skillet over medium heat. Once the oil is hot, add 1 tbsp of batter per pancake to the skillet. Cook until the tops stop bubbling and flip, then cook the other side. Continue cooking until the batter is used up, adding additional coconut oil to the skillet as needed. Transfer the cooked pancakes to a plate and cover to keep warm until you're ready to serve.

Spinach Quiche

Number of servings: 4

Ingredients:

6 large eggs
2 cups baby spinach leaves, chopped
½ of a small red onion, diced
1 clove of garlic, minced
½ cup of coconut milk
½ tsp baking powder
salt and black pepper, to taste

Preparation:

Start by preheating your oven to 350 F. While the oven is heating, whisk together the coconut milk and eggs in a large bowl. Add the remaining ingredients, whisking well to combine. Lightly oil a 9" pie dish and pour in the egg mixture. Place the quiche in the oven and bake for about half an hour or until the quiche is cooked through at the center. Remove from the oven, allow to rest for a few minutes, slice and serve.

Cucumber – Blueberry Smoothie

Number of servings: 2 – 4, depending on serving size

Ingredients:

2 large cucumbers, peeled and diced
1 cup frozen blueberries
1 cup of coconut milk
juice of 1 lemon or lime

Preparation:

This is perhaps the easiest recipe in the entire book. Just put all of the ingredients in a blender, blend until smooth and serve.

Cranberry – Almond Bread

Number of servings: varies

Ingredients:

3 large eggs
¾ cup almond butter
½ cup dried cranberries
¼ cup dried apricots, chopped
¼ cup pumpkin seeds
¼ cup sesame seeds
¼ cup sunflower seeds
¼ cup sliced almonds, plus a little extra for topping
¼ cup arrowroot powder
2 tbsp olive oil, plus a little extra for greasing the pan
1 tsp salt
¼ tsp baking soda
a little almond flour, for dusting

Preparation:

Preheat your oven to 350 F. Add the oil, eggs and almond butter to a large bowl and blend until smooth with a hand blender or egg beater. In a separate, small bowl, mix together the arrowroot powder, salt and baking soda; add the arrowroot mixture to the wet ingredients and mix until well combined. Stir in the dried fruits, seeds and nuts.

Oil a loaf pan with olive oil and dust with a little almond

flour. Pour the batter into the prepared loaf pan and sprinkle with sliced almonds. Place the pan in the oven and bake for 45 – 50 minutes, or until a knife inserted into the center of the loaf comes out clean. Remove the loaf from the oven and allow to cool for at least one hour before slicing and serving.

Irish Soda Bread

Number of servings: varies

Ingredients:

3 cups almond flour
2 eggs
½ cup raisins
2 tbsp honey
2 tbsp apple cider vinegar
1 ½ tsp baking soda
¼ tsp baking soda
a pinch of caraway seeds

Preparation:

Preheat your oven to 350 F. Combine the almond flour, raisins, salt and baking soda in a large bowl and mix well. In a separate, smaller bowl, whisk together the eggs, honey and vinegar. Add the wet ingredients to the dry ingredients and mix well.

Transfer the dough to a piece of parchment paper and shape into a roughly 8" circular loaf. Score the top of the loaf with a serrated knife in a cross pattern. Sprinkle the top with caraway seeds. Transfer the loaf (still on the parchment paper) to a baking sheet and bake for 20 minutes. Turn off the heat, but leave the loaf in the oven for another 10 minutes before removing. Allow the soda bread to cool for at least 30 minutes. Slice and serve with butter and/or preserves.

Desserts

Chocolate - Avocado Mousse

Number of servings: 8

Ingredients:

The mousse:
4 ripe avocados, peeled and seeded
10 dates, pitted
4 tbsp honey
2 tbsp cacao powder
½ cup pomegranate seeds
The crust:
1 ½ cups walnuts
2 tbsp maple syrup
a pinch of salt

Preparation:

The crust will take longer to make, so start with this part. Add the walnuts to a food processor and grind into small pieces. Add the salt and maple syrup until it forms a coarse dough-like consistency. Add about 2 tbsp of the mixture to 8 ramekins and press into the bottom to form a crust. Transfer the ramekins to the refrigerator to allow the crust to harden.

Place the avocadoes in a food processor, along with the dates, cacao powder and honey. Process the ingredients until completely they are completely smooth. Transfer the mouse into a piping bag (you can make your own by adding the mousse to a ziplock bag and cutting off one corner).

Remove the ramekins from the refrigerator and pipe the mousse into the ramekins. Return the ramekins to the refrigerator and chill for at least 1 hour. Serve cold, garnished with pomegranate seeds.

Chocolate – Cranberry Pie

Number of servings: 6 - 8

Ingredients:

The crust:
2 cups almond flour
1 egg
2 tbsp coconut oil
½ tsp salt
The filling and toppings:
1 lb frozen cranberries (about 2 cups)
½ cup coconut milk
8 ounces dark chocolate (70% cocoa)
½ cup sugar

Preparation:

Start by preheating your oven to 375 F while you make the crust. Add all of the ingredients to a blender and process until they form a crumbly dough (much like traditional pastry dough). Lightly grease a 9" pie dish and transfer the dough into the prepared dish. Use your hands to press the dough evenly over the bottom of the pie dish.
Place the crust in the oven and bake for about 15 minutes, or until it turns golden brown and flaky.
Remove the crust from the oven and allow it to cool to room temperature.
You can start making the filling while the crust bakes.

Pour the coconut milk into a small saucepan and bring to a boil over medium – high heat. Once it reaches a boil, remove from heat at once and add the chocolate and 1/4 cup of sugar. Stir continuously until the chocolate melts completely and is combined with the coconut milk. Pour the filling into the cooled pie shell and transfer the pie to the refrigerator. Chill for at least 2 hours and for as long as 24 hours to allow the filling to solidify.

Preheat your oven to 375 F. Once the oven is hot, spread the cranberries on a baking sheet, sprinkle with ¼ cup of sugar and bake for about 10 minutes, stirring once or twice to prevent them from sticking. When the cranberries are soft and starting to blister, remove from heat and transfer them to a bowl. Refrigerate the cranberries for at least 1 hour. Spoon the cooled cranberries on top of the pie, slice and serve.

Paleolithic Style Coconut Cream Pie

Number of servings: 6 – 8

Ingredients:

The crust:
3 large eggs
2 ounces dark chocolate (85% - 90% cacao)
¾ cup coconut flour
½ cup coconut flakes
¼ cup coconut oil
2 tbsp cold water (or more, if necessary)
2 tbsp coconut sugar (or sugar, if you can't find coconut sugar)
1 tsp vanilla extract
¼ tsp baking soda
¼ tsp salt
The filling:
4 egg yolks from large eggs
2 cans (14 ounces) coconut milk
2/3 cup creamed coconut
2/3 cup coconut sugar (or sugar, if you can't find coconut sugar)
9 tbsp arrowroot powder
1 tsp vanilla extract
¼ tsp salt
The topping:
½ cup coconut flakes
dark chocolate shavings

Preparation:

Preheat your oven to 325 F. Add the coconut flakes and coconut flour to a food processor and pulse until thoroughly combined. Whisk together the coconut oil, eggs, salt, coconut sugar, vanilla extract and baking soda in a medium sized bowl. Add the egg mixture to the dry ingredients in the food processor and pulse until the mixture forms a crumbly, pastry dough – like mixture. Add the water very slowly until the dough comes together and is slightly moist.

Spread the dough with your hands in a 9" pie dish to form a crust. Place in the oven and bake the crust for 15 minutes, or until it is golden brown. Remove from the oven and allow it to cool completely. Melt the chocolate in a microwave or in a double boiler. Brush the cooled pie shell with melted chocolate. Transfer the pie shell to the refrigerator to allow the chocolate to harden.

Add ice cubes and cold water to a large bowl and set it aside. In a medium sized bowl, whisk the egg yolks and set aside. Add the coconut milk, creamed coconut, coconut sugar, salt and vanilla extract to a saucepan and bring to a simmer. Cook for about 10 minutes, whisking constantly to prevent separation. The mixture will thicken as it cooks. Whisk ¼ of the coconut milk mixture into the egg yolks, then add the remainder of the mixture and whisk well to combine.

Return the coconut milk and egg mixture to the

saucepan and cook over medium- high heat, whisking constantly until it thickens and bubbles start to form in the center of the custard (about 10 minutes). Pour the custard into a medium sized bowl and transfer the bowl into the ice bath. Allow the custard to cool for 30 – 40 minutes, whisking occasionally. Add the arrowroot powder and whisk until combined and slightly thickened. Place a sheet of plastic wrap on the surface of the custard (this will prevent a skin from forming on your custard) and transfer to the refrigerator. Chill for at least 4 hours and for as long as 24 hours to allow the custard to thicken.

Toast the coconut flakes in a dry skillet over medium heat, stirring occasionally and set aside. Remove the pie shell from the refrigerator and fill with the custard, using a spatula to spread it evenly. Return the pie to the refrigerator and chill for at least 3 hours. Garnish with toasted coconut flakes and dark chocolate shavings, slice and serve.

Pineapple – Coconut Frozen Custard

Number of servings: varies depending on serving sizes

Ingredients:

¾ cup finely chopped fresh pineapple
1 (14 ounce) can coconut milk
4 egg yolks
¼ cup pineapple juice
3 tbsp honey
1 tbsp vanilla extract

Preparation:

Note: You'll need an ice cream maker to make this recipe.
Add the pineapple juice, coconut milk, vanilla extract and honey to a medium sized saucepan and bring to a simmer over medium – low heat.

While the coconut milk and pineapple juice mixture is heating, whisk the egg yolks in a small bowl until they're frothy. Pour ¼ of the hot coconut milk and pineapple juice mixture into the eggs, whisking as you add it in. Pour this mixture into the saucepan and whisk to combine. Return the mixture to a simmer, whisking constantly until the mixture thickens slightly – this will take about 5 minutes.

Transfer to a bowl and refrigerate until cool. Once the

mixture is cooled, pour into an electric ice cream maker and proceed according to the manufacturer's directions. A few minutes before it's done, add the chopped pineapple. When the machine completes the process, you can eat your frozen custard right away, but it will be fairly soft. For a harder ice cream, freeze the custard for a few hours before serving.

About the Recipes Contained in this Book

These recipes were selected to be suitable for the diet and lifestyle discussed in this book. Although we create our own recipes, we also do like to give credit to the amazing chefs who inspired our work. Some recipes may be adapted from other popular recipes on the internet or other sources. We would like to give credit and thanks for this.

The book presents our favorites and the recipes we feel fit the topic best in order to provide the highest quality experience for our highly valued readers.

Paleolithic Cookbook Conclusion

There's no getting around the fact that like any kind of diet, the Paleolithic diet does limit what you can eat in certain ways – but as you can see from the wide variety of recipes in this cookbook, you definitely don't have to feel deprived when you take up this diet. However, there are some very important differences between this and the fad diets which seem to come and go in a matter of weeks or months.

Unlike fad diets, the Paleolithic diet isn't just a diet; it's a lifestyle which ideally incorporates diet and exercise into a harmonious whole which leads to better health and meals which are every bit as delicious – if not more so – than anything you were eating before. In fact, many of the recipes here are simply healthier variations on dishes which you already enjoy. Once you get used to living without processed foods and going light on the dairy and sugar, you won't miss eating a conventional modern diet one bit!

Using the recipes and ideas found in this book as a sort of template, you can and should feel free to experiment in the kitchen. Substitute grains with healthier choices like spaghetti squash or zucchini noodles for pasta and almond flour for wheat flour, reduce the amount of sugar you eat and wherever possible, replace it with honey or maple syrup and you'll be well on your way to coming up with some new, Paleolithic-friendly, healthy and most important of all, delicious culinary creations of your very own. There are only a few rules in the Paleolithic diet and aside from these, your imagination is the only limit to what you can come up with!

Section 2: Grain Free Recipes Introduction

There's something absolutely delicious about a freshly baked loaf of bread, a crispy waffle, or a tasty cake hot out of the oven! These foods all have one thing in common: they're made with grain or wheat flour. Cooking with wheat flour and grain is something that everyone does, and it produces a whole lot of delicious foods.

Unfortunately for many, grain and wheat are things that they cannot enjoy. Gluten intolerance can be a serious problem for many people, and they are unable to eat foods that contain lots of grain or wheat. When they do, they have serious digestive problems, or their body can react strongly and negatively to the gluten in the grain that they are eating.

Gluten has been linked to a number of problems. Interestingly enough, the body often sees gluten as being a foreign substance that it can't process. While gluten is commonly found in the food we eat, it wasn't always part of our diet. The human body can't always process this gooey, sticky protein easily, and it can be a bit hard on the body if you happen to be sensitive to it. Even those without celiac problems may not be able to handle the gluten, as their bodies react to the "foreign substance" by attacking it with antibodies.

Cutting grain out of your diet can help to reduce your risk of health problems, especially if you have celiac disorder or other gluten-sensitive problems. However, even for those that don't have these health problems, it may be a good idea to cut gluten out of your diet. Many people don't have celiac disease, and yet they still experience the drawbacks of eating gluten.

In an article in the New Zealand edition of Stuff magazine, an article by a world-renowned expert on food allergies, Dr. Rodney Ford, states, "Gluten causes tiredness, anxiety and stress. The medical world accepts it can damage the gut, but it can also damage the brain, skin and nerves. Until now, many of these illnesses have been blamed on everything from stress at home to other medical conditions, including depression." [1]

Cutting gluten out of your life isn't just something you can do to prevent celiac problems, but it can be good for your health. Many holistic doctors and therapists will recommend cutting it from your diet, as it carries the risk of causing negative side effects.

Did you know that eliminating grain and gluten can be beneficial to your body? The benefits include:

- Reduced risk of IBS or other digestive problems
- Less chance of becoming fatigued, depressed, nauseous, or developing stomach cramps

- Boost in your energy levels
- Reduced body fat percentage
- Increase in lean muscle tissue
- Lowered blood pressure
- Improved mood and sense of wellbeing
- As you can see, there are many great reasons to cut grain from your diet!

"But," you may say, "all of my favorite foods are made with grain! How can I cut grain out of my diet and still enjoy the food I'm eating?"

Don't worry about it! In this book, you'll find plenty of delicious recipes that you can make without needing to use grain, and you can whip up your favorite dishes and still make them gluten-free. You'll have to spend a bit of money to stock your house with some ingredients you probably don't have right now, but you'll be amazed at how many delicious foods you can make without using grain.

Enjoy the book, and happy grain-free cooking!

Tasty Grain Free Recipes

Grain Free Breaded Chicken

There's nothing like some breaded chicken to kick off your lunch in style, but bread crumbs have wheat, right? Here is a quick and easy recipe you can use to make breaded chicken without the bread...

Ingredients

For this dish, you will need:

1 large chicken breast
1 cup of almond flour
½ cup of Kraft's Parmesan Cheese
Thyme
Basil
Oregano
½ cup of butter
Red or crushed chili pepper
Garlic powder
Salt and pepper, to taste

Preparation:

To begin, slice the chicken breast into steaks -- preferably about three steaks from each half of the breast. You should have about 6 medium steaks from the breast.

Preheat your oven to about 350 F. Use a bit of butter to grease the bottom of a baking tray.

In a bowl, combine the almond flour with the Parmesan cheese. Sprinkle in about a teaspoon each of basil, thyme, and oregano, and add in a pinch of crushed red pepper for some spice. A teaspoon of garlic powder will help to add the flavor you want, and a bit of salt and black pepper will round out the flavors.

In a saucepan, melt the butter. Dip the chicken steaks into the butter, ensuring that the entire surface of the chicken is coated well. Roll the buttered strips in the almond flour, and make sure that they are properly coated with the flour mixture.

Place the steaks onto your baking tray, laying them as flat as possible. Transfer the tray into the oven, and let the steaks cook for about 20 minutes. They should be a wonderful golden brown, and they will be absolutely delightful to eat! (Check to make sure that they aren't pink in the center, as that's a sign that the chicken is undercooked.)

Sesame Seed Chicken Fried Steak

Want to eat that Southern-style chicken fried steak that your mama used to make you? This simple recipe won't make it exactly like the regular steak, but it's as close as you'll get while on a gluten-free diet!

Ingredients

For this dish, you will need:
4 large steaks, sliced fairly thin
2 eggs
½ cup of almond flour
1/3 cup of sesame seeds
1/4 cup of flax seeds
Chicken bouillon powder
Basil
Bay leaves
Garlic powder
Salt and black pepper, to taste

Preparation:

To begin, place a pan on the stove to heat, and add in enough oil to deep fry your breaded steak. Let the oil heat as you go about preparing the rest of the meal.

Crack the 2 eggs into a bowl, and beat them vigorously to combine the egg and yolk. Add a pinch of salt into the eggs.

Combine the almond flour, a pinch each of chicken bouillon, garlic powder, salt, and pepper, and the flax seeds in a bowl. Add the sesame seeds into the bowl, and crush three bay leaves in your hands to add them into the mix. Use a fork to stir the dry ingredients together, and make sure that they're properly combined before moving on.

Dip each steak into the eggs, and roll the dipped meat into the flour and seed mixture. Make sure that the entire surface of the meat has been properly coated. If you want to really get the flour coating on right, you can roll the meat in the flour before dipping it into the egg, and roll it a second time after dipping to ensure that the layer of flour is very thick.

Place the steaks in the hot oil one at a time, and cook them until they are golden brown. Remove them from the pan once they are properly cooked, and place them on a plate with paper towels beneath and above them to soak up the oil.

Let the steaks sit until they are all cooked, transfer onto a plate, and serve.

Gluten and Sugar-Free Gingerbread Cake

Want a delicious dessert to make your Christmas celebrations complete? This gluten and sugar-free gingerbread cake will have all of the flavor of the holiday, but with none of the unhealthy nutrients that you're trying to avoid!

Ingredients:

For this cake, you will need:
½ cup of coconut flour
1 cup of amaranth flour
1 cup of buckwheat flour
2 tablespoons of flax meal (For those who want the non-vegan version of this cake, use 2 eggs instead of the flax meal. It will make the cake a bit fluffier, and will help to round out the flavors nicely.)
2 ½ teaspoons of baking soda
Ground cinnamon
Ground ginger
Ground cloves
Ground nutmeg
Salt
Water
¾ cup of agave nectar
¾ cup of molasses
Canola oil
Fresh ginger
Lemon zest

Preparation:

To begin, turn on the oven and let it heat to 350 F. As the oven is heating, prepare the cake.

Combine the coconut flour, amaranth flour, buckwheat flour, and baking soda in a bowl. Add in 2 teaspoons of cinnamon, the same amount of ground ginger, half a teaspoon each of cloves, salt, and nutmeg, and a teaspoon or two of lemon zest. Stir the ingredients well to combine.

In a separate bowl, combine the flax meal with a few tablespoons of water, and stir in the agave, the molasses, ¾ of a cup of canola oil, and a couple of teaspoons of the grated fresh ginger. Mix these ingredients together well, and pour them into the bowl with the dry ingredients. Stir the wet and dry ingredients together to make the batter for the cake, and add about a cup of boiling water to your final batter.

Once the water has been properly mixed in with the rest of the ingredients, pour the cake batter into a buttered baking pan. Place the pan into the oven, and let it cook for about 40 minutes.

You'll find that a toothpick or knife inserted into the center of the cake will come out clean, and it will let you know that your cake is ready to enjoy.

Cut once the cake has cooled a bit, and serve.

Gluten Free Waffles

There's nothing like a heaping stack of waffles to get your morning started the right way, but your regular waffles are loaded with grain and gluten. These delicious grain-free waffles will be the perfect breakfast, and it will help you to enjoy what you're eating without having to worry about adding grain to your diet.

Ingredients

For this dish, you will need:
1 cup of rice flour
1/3 cups of potato starch (not all cornstarch products are gluten-free)
3 tablespoons of tapioca flour
1 ½ teaspoons of baking powder
½ teaspoon of baking soda
Salt
Xantham gum
Buttermilk
Sugar substitute
2 eggs
Canola oil
2 cups of water

Preparation:

To begin, heat your waffle iron. It takes about 5 to 10 minutes for the waffle iron to heat -- depending on the brand -- so make sure that it's heating as you go about preparing the waffles.

Mix the rice flour, potato starch, tapioca flour, baking soda, and baking powder together in a bowl. Add in about half a teaspoon of salt, and the same amount of xantham gum. Mix the dry ingredients together, and be sure that they are properly combined before moving on to the next step.

Crack the two eggs into another bowl, and add in the water. Add about 3 tablespoons of the oil, and mix the ingredients together well. Stir them in with the dry ingredients, and mix until you get the waffle batter you want. The batter will be a bit thick, so add buttermilk to produce the desired consistency for the waffle batter. Make sure that there are no lumps.

Use some spray cooking oil to grease the waffle iron, or use regular oil on a paper towel to cover the iron with a thin layer of oil. Pour the batter into the heated iron, and close the lid. Watch the waffle iron until the light turns off, and use a fork to remove the cooked waffle from the waffle maker.

Serve while hot, and enjoy the delicious, crunchy waffles!

Buckwheat Pancakes

For those of you who just can't stay away from those flapjacks, this pancake recipe will be the perfect grain-free solution for you! You'll still be able to have a tall stack of delicious pancakes, but without worrying about gluten or grain.

Ingredients

For this dish, you will need:
1 ½ cups of buckwheat flour
3 tablespoons of sugar (use sugar alternative for a low-sugar meal)
Salt
1 teaspoon of baking soda
Unsalted butter
1 egg
Buttermilk

Preparation:

To begin, place a frying pan on the stove to heat. Make sure that it has been properly heated before placing the batter onto the pan, so give it time to warm up as you make the pancakes.

Mix the flour, sugar, and baking soda together in a bowl. Add in about a teaspoon of salt. Stir the ingredients well to combine.

Crack your egg in another bowl, and beat to combine the yolk and white.

Melt the butter in a saucepan or the microwave, and pour the melted butter over the flour mixture -- stirring as you pour. Add the egg into the mix, and pour in about a cup of buttermilk as well. Stir the batter together, and you'll have a fairly thick mixture. Keep pouring in buttermilk until your pancakes have reached the desired consistency, and stir to ensure that there are no lumps.

Once the batter has been prepared, pour it into a pitcher or an empty ketchup bottle. Gently pour or squeeze the batter onto your heated pan, which you will have coated with a bit of oil to butter to prevent the pancakes from sticking.

Cook until the top of the pancake is riddled with bubbles, and flip it over to cook on the other side for about 20 seconds.

Once the batter has been used up, you'll have a delicious stack of healthy buckwheat pancakes that are grain-free and fairly low calorie!

Grain-Free Cornbread

You can't have chili beans without some delicious cornbread, and there are so many other dishes that won't be complete without this delicious savory baked bread. Don't worry about it being high in grain, as we've substituted the ingredients in the bread for grain-free ones!

Ingredients

For this dish, you will need:
1 ½ cups of cornmeal
1 cup of millet flour
1 cup of rice flour
2 eggs
Water
Vegetable oil
¼ cup of sugar
1 tablespoon of baking powder
Salt

Preparation:

To begin, heat your oven to about 400 degrees. This way, it will be hot enough to cook the bread, but it won't be so hot that the bread will burn.

Use a bit of butter to grease a 9x9 baking dish, and set it aside as you prepare the bread.

In a bowl, crack and beat the eggs vigorously to combine the yolk and egg white. Heat 1 ½ cups of water until they are lukewarm, and add them into the eggs. Drop in ¼ cup of canola or vegetable oil, and mix the ingredients well until they are properly blended.

In a separate bowl, mix the millet flour, rice flour, and cornmeal together. Add in the white sugar, the baking powder, and about a teaspoon of salt. Make sure that the dry ingredients are all mixed together properly, and hollow out a hole in the center of the bowl.

Pour the wet ingredients into the hollowed center of the flour mixture, and use a whisk to stir the ingredients together properly. Whisk and stir until you are sure that there are no lumps, which could take a few minutes.

Once you're sure there are no lumps, pour the batter into the greased baking pan. Place the pan into the oven, and let it cook for about 20 minutes. You can tell that it's cooked by pressing on the surface of the bread. If it's properly done, the corn bread will spring back up when you press gently on it.

Remove from the oven, let the cornbread cool for a few minutes, and serve while still warm.

Curried Quinoa

This delicious side dish is made without any grain, which means that you can eat it whenever you want! The quinoa is a much lower-calorie alternative to rice, but it will be a delicious alternative that will make the dish absolutely fantastic!

Ingredients:

For this dish, you will need:
1 cup of quinoa
Olive oil
1 onion
Garlic
2 cups of chicken broth
Curry powder
Ancho chili powder
Salt and pepper

Preparation:

To begin, place a skillet on the stove to heat. Bring it to medium heat, and pour a couple of tablespoons of olive oil into the pan.

Chop the onion very finely, and add between 3 and 5 cloves of garlic -- depending on your flavor preference. Cook the aromatics in the oil, leaving them in the pan for about 5 minutes to ensure that you have extracted the flavor from them. Add the quinoa into the pan, and cook the seed in the oil until it is lightly toasted.

Once you're done cooking the quinoa, pour the chicken broth into the pan. Cover the pan, and let the broth heat until it begins to boil. Stir in about a tablespoon each of the curry powder and Mexican chili powder, and cover the pan once again.

Turn the heat down to let the quinoa simmer, and let it cook on low heat for about 25 minutes. The quinoa should be soft and tasty, and you can add a bit of salt and pepper to add the flavor you want for the dish. (Serve as the starch with nearly any protein, and it will be a delicious companion for your meal!)

Roasted Almond Cookies

Want to enjoy a delicious dessert without getting into the grain-loaded cookie jar? These cookies are quick and easy to make, and you'll find that they're the perfect grain-free solution to help you stay true to your gluten-free diet!

Ingredients:

For this dish, you will need:
1 cup of raw almonds
½ cup of maple syrup
1 cup of oat flour
Almond extract

Preparation:

Preheat the oven to about 275 F, which will be hot enough to toast the almonds.

Place the cup of almonds onto a baking sheet, and put them in the oven. Let them heat until they become golden brown and are releasing a delightful scent, which will take about 40 minutes. Be careful that they don't burn.

Once the almonds are cooked, remove them from the oven and set them aside to cool. After they have cooled down enough, run them through your food processor to produce a fine almond flour.

Mix the flour in a bowl together with the oat flour, maple syrup, and almond extract.

Turn the heat of the oven up to 350 F, and let it heat.

As the oven is heating, use your hands to form the dough into 6 balls. Press the balls gently to flatten them a bit, until they are about half an inch thick. Place the cookies onto a greased baking sheet, and put the sheet in the oven.

Let the cookies bake for about 12 minutes, but keep a close eye on them because the edges can burn very quickly. They will become browned and crisp around the edges of the cookie, and that's how you'll know that they're done.

Remove them from the oven, let them cool, and enjoy!

Grain-Free Zucchini Bread

Most people think of banana bread or carrot cake as being the only vegetable-laden desserts that you can make, but you'll find that zucchini bread will be a delicious alternative that will be just as healthy and tasty! Thanks to the grain-free recipe, you won't have to worry about the gluten.

Ingredients:

For this dish, you will need:
1 cup of teff flour
1 cup of buckwheat flour
Baking soda
Salt
Baking powder
3 eggs
Lemon zest
Cinnamon
1 cup of apple sauce
½ cup of maple syrup
Coconut oil
Vanilla extract
2 cups of grated zucchini
1 cup of raisins and almonds mixed

Preparation:

To begin, turn on your oven and pre-heat it to about 350 degrees. As it's heating, move on to the next step.

Mix the buckwheat and teff flours together in a bowl, and add in a tablespoon of cinnamon, a teaspoon of salt and lemon zest each, 2 teaspoons of the baking soda, and ¼ teaspoon of baking powder. Stir well to ensure that the ingredients are properly combined before moving on.

In a separate bowl, combine the apple sauce and maple syrup together, and crack the three eggs into the bowl. Beat well to mix the ingredients, and add two teaspoons of vanilla extract and a tablespoon of coconut oil into the bowl. Stir well to mix.

Once the wet ingredients are properly mixed, pour the dry ingredients into the bowl. Stir well or use an electric mixer to combine the ingredients, and stir until there are no more lumps. Pour the zucchini into the batter, and add the raisins and almonds as well. Mix to distribute these ingredients.

Pour the batter into a greased baking pan, which should have a bit of butter along the bottom to help make the cake tasty. Put the pan into the oven, and let it cook for about 50 minutes. The cake will take longer to cook than your average flour cake, but you'll know that it's done when a toothpick or knife inserted into the center of the cake comes out clean.

Remove the cake from the oven, let cool for a few minutes, cut, and serve!

Apple Cobbler

Not quite the same as Apple Crumble, this Apple Cobbler recipe is the perfect grain-free breakfast treat! It will be crunchy, flavorful, and delightful, but it won't have any of the gluten that you're trying so hard to avoid.

Ingredients

For this dish, you will need:
6 apples
1 can of cranberry sauce
Brown sugar
1 cup of steel-cut oats
Cinnamon
Soy milk
Butter

Preparation:

To begin, peel and cut the apples. You will want to make them small slices, easy enough to fit into your mouth without being too small.

Preheat the oven to about 350 F once the apples are done. Grease a baking tray with a bit of butter, and set it aside as you move on.

Combine the apples and the cranberry sauce in a bowl, and add in 2 or 3 tablespoons of the brown sugar. Add ¼ cup of soy milk, and mix the ingredients well to ensure that they are properly combined.

Melt a bit of butter on the stove, and pour the butter over the top of the oats. Toss the oats to coat them evenly with the butter.

Place the apple mixture into the pan, and cover it with a top layer of oats. Place the pan into the oven, and let it cook for about 35 or 40 minutes. You'll see that the oats turn a pleasant golden brown, and the juices released by the apple and cranberry sauce will bubble nicely.

Remove from the oven, let cool for a few minutes, and serve as the perfect healthy breakfast!

Breakfast Cereal Sans Gluten

A healthy breakfast cereal can be the perfect thing to get your morning started the right way, as it will provide you with slow-burning carbs that will give you energy all day long. This breakfast cereal will be perfect, as it comes without grain and will give you that energy boost you need for the long day ahead.

Ingredients:

For this dish, you will need:
½ cup of quinoa
½ cup of buckwheat groats
1 cup of brown basmati rice
½ cup of millet
½ cup of flax seeds
½ cup of sesame seeds
½ cup of cornmeal
½ cup of amaranth

Preparation:

To begin, place the basmati rice into a blender or grinder, and grind until you have produced a coarse rice flour. Empty the rice into a bowl.

Grind or blend all of the other ingredients, and you will end up with a mixture of various flours -- none of which will be wheat or grain flour, of course.

To prepare the cereal, put 4 cups of water into a pan to boil on the stove. Once the water is boiling, add in about a cup of the cereal mixture and a pinch of salt. Add a tablespoon or two of milk powder, and let the ingredients cook until they have thickened.

To add some flavor, add in a bit of cinnamon, some butter, and a tablespoon of sugar. You'll find that these ingredients will sweeten the cereal, and a bit of milk will help to make it more edible.

The cereal mixture will take about 20 minutes to cook, and you should keep the heat low to prevent it from burning. After 20 minutes has passed, scoop into a bowl, let cool for a minute, and enjoy!

Rice Stuffing

Need to stuff that Thanksgiving turkey but don't want to use bread? This rice turkey or chicken stuffing will be the perfect thing for you! It's tasty, subtle, and easy to make, and it will enable you to give your turkey the right filling.

Ingredients:

For this dish, you will need:
2 cups of white rice
Water
Chicken bouillon
1 onion
Butter
Garlic
1 celery stalk
Parsley
Salt
Sage
Thyme
Pepper, to taste

Preparation:

To begin, you will need to dice the onions as fine as you can. Make sure to chop the onions very small.

Place a pot on the stove to heat, and add about a tablespoon of butter into the bottom of the pan. Once the butter has melted, add the onions into the mixture. Let the onions fry for a minute, and chop the garlic as you do so. Add about 5 cloves of garlic -- chopped fine -- into the pan, and fry the garlic along with the onions.

Once the onions have begun to brown around the edges, add the uncooked rice into the pan. You will want to cook the rice until it shows signs of beginning to burn, and the grains will become slightly browned. At this point, add the 2 cups of water into the pan, and cover it.

Once the rice begins to simmer, add a tablespoon or two of chicken bouillon into the pan. Dice the celery stalk, and drop the pieces into the pan. Sprinkle parsley, salt, sage, thyme, and all the pepper you want into the rice.

The simmering water will cook the rice in about 20 minutes, but keep a close eye on it. once the level of the rice rises above the water level, you only have about 5 to 7 more minutes until the rice is completely cooked. Make sure the rice doesn't burn, and don't let it cook all the way. The rice should still be a bit crunchy when you turn it off.

Once the rice is cooked, remove it from the pan, let it cool, and use it to stuff your turkey. The partially cooked rice will finish cooking as the turkey cooks, and it will come out soft and fluffy!

Gluten Free Irish Shortbread

There's nothing like a good piece of Irish shortbread to eat after your Irish beef stew, and you'll find that a hearty piece of this bread will go down nicely. The best part about this bread: it's made without gluten or wheat!

Ingredients

For this dish, you will need:
2 cups of butter
2 cups of rye flour
1 cup of corn flour
2 cups of brown sugar

Preparation:

To begin, heat the oven to 300 degrees. Take the time to grease two baking pans, or use grease paper to prevent a mess.

Soften the butter in a double boiler, or leave it at room temperature for an hour to make it easier to mash. Use a fork to mix the sugar into the butter, and combine it until it is creamy and blended. Add the corn flour and the rye flour, and combine into a nice dough.

Divide the dough that you have into two portions, and press each portion of dough into the pans that you have prepared. Use the fork to prick some shallow holes, dividing the bread into individual portions. You can sprinkle a bit of sugar to make it decorative.

Place the baking pans into the oven, and let them cook for about an hour. You'll find that the bread can cook in as little time as 45 minutes, so keep an eye on it. You may notice that the edges of the bread are getting browned, and the top will be nicely golden.

Cut the bread into individual pieces while it is still warm, and enjoy!

Asian Sesame Noodles

If you love the taste of the Orient, this will definitely be the dish for you. These tasty noodles are grain-free, but they're absolutely delightful! With the right ingredients added to this dish, you'll have everything you need to get your Oriental on!

Ingredients

For this dish, you will need:
400 grams of Gluten-free noodles
Sesame oil
2 carrots
Garlic
Fresh ginger root
1 onion
½ head of cabbage
½ pepper
1 sprig of cilantro
Almond butter
Gluten-free soy sauce

Preparation:

To begin, you'll need to put a pot of water on the stove to boil. Add about 3 cups of water per 100 grams of noodles, and give it a few minutes to boil.

As the water is heating up, dice the ginger, garlic, and onions. You can use as much garlic as you want, but add no more than a teaspoon of fresh ginger root. Julienne the carrots, the bell pepper, and the cabbage, making the slices as thin as possible.

Place a wok on the stove to heat, and pour in a few tablespoons of sesame oil. Once the oil is hot, drop in the ginger, garlic, and onions. Stir fry the ingredients for a few minutes, and add in the carrots. Once the carrots have begun to soften, add in the peppers and the cabbage. Cook for just 3 minutes, and add the soy sauce into the mixture.

Place the noodles in the water to cook, and keep a close eye on them. You don't want them to overcook, as they'll be quite unpleasant. Make sure that they're al dente, and remove them from the stove. Drain the water, run cold water over the noodles, and throw the noodles into the wok.

Stir fry the noodles with the other ingredients, adding a tablespoon of almond butter, 2 tablespoons of soy sauce, and ½ tablespoon of sesame oil to flavor the noodles. Cook until the liquid has all been eliminated from the wok, leaving you with a dry, slightly fried noodle dish.

Serve the noodles onto two plates, chop the cilantro to sprinkle on top of the noodles, and serve with chopsticks and your favorite Chinese hot sauce.

Shrimp Cakes

Want to enjoy some seafood, but can't eat gluten? These gluten-free shrimp cakes are an absolute delight, and they'll help you to get a lot more protein in your diet. They're fairly easy to make, but they're definitely a delicious meal that will be ideal for anyone on a weight loss diet.

Ingredients

For this dish, you will need:
1 pound of shrimp
1 red bell pepper
2 cloves of garlic
Scallions
Lime juice
Sea salt
Chipotle
1 egg
½ cup of almond flour
Grapeseed or peanut
½ cup of chopped cilantro

Preparation:

To begin, peel and de-vein the shrimp. This can be a lengthy process, so be prepared to spend at least 20 minutes in this activity.

Once the shrimp has been prepared, throw them into

the blender or food processor. Press the pulse button until the shrimp has been chopped fine, and remove the shrimp from the blender.

Pour the shrimp into a bowl, and add a teaspoon of sea salt, the cilantro, and ¼ teaspoon of chipotle. Crack the egg into the bowl, and mix it well to combine.

Dice the scallions, the garlic, and the bell pepper, making sure that they are very finely chopped. Add them into the bowl, and stir to mix properly. Add the lime juice for the finishing flavor touches.

Use your hands to form the ingredients into balls, which you will dip into the almond flour to coat them thoroughly as you flatten them into patties.

Place a skillet on the stove to heat, and add enough oil to fry the patties. Place four of the patties into the skillet at a time, and cook for about 5 minutes. Turn the patty onto its other side, and cook it until that side is also browned.

Remove the cooked patties from the pan, and place them on a paper towel to drain as you cook the rest. You should obtain about 12 patties from this mixture.

Enjoy with a simple marinara sauce, or just pour some of your favorite hot sauce over the patties to make them taste delicious!

Stuffed Bell Peppers

This dish is made with a rice stuffing that will be absolutely divine, not to mention free of gluten. If you want to enjoy a delicious stuffed bell pepper, this is a recipe that you must try!

Ingredients:

For this dish, you will need:
6 green bell peppers
Diced green chilies
1 pound of ground beef
1 onion
5 cloves of garlic
1 cup of rice
Cumin
Cilantro
Chili powder
Sea salt

Preparation:

To begin, place a pan on the stove to heat. Pour a tablespoon of oil into the bottom of the pan, and dice one of the cloves of garlic. Cook the garlic until it's nicely browned, and add the rice into the pan. Once the rice is toasted, pour 1 cup of water into the pan. Cover it and cook on low heat until the rice is done. Remove from the heat and set aside.

Dice the onion and the rest of the garlic very finely, and place a skillet on the stove to heat. With a bit of oil in the bottom of the pan, sauté the garlic and onions for a few minutes. Add the ground beef into the pan, and cook it until it's well done. Add ½ can of diced green chilies 3 minutes before the meat is done, and cook them with the meat. Once you have turned off the meat, add in a teaspoon of cumin, ½ cup of diced fresh cilantro, a teaspoon of chili powder, and a tablespoon of sea salt.

Take the ground beef mixture and add it into the pan with the rice. Mix well to combine, and add salt and pepper as desired.

Use a knife to score around the top of the bell pepper, and pull off the top to extract the seeds. Wash the peppers thoroughly to remove any remaining seeds.

Heat the oven to 350 F.

Use a spoon to scoop the rice and beef mixture into the bell peppers, stuffing them completely full. Remove the seeds from the tops of the bell peppers, and place the tops back on the peppers. Place the bell peppers on a tray, and place the tray in the oven.

Let the peppers cook for about 45 minutes to an hour, and they will be ready to eat!

Gluten-Free Turkey Club

This is a delicious sandwich that you can make all on your own, and you'll be able to use gluten-free bread to slap together this quick and easy meal. You can used gluten-free bread that you bought from the store, or you can make your own loaf of gluten-free nut bread. This recipe will just tell you how to make the perfect sandwich, but there's a recipe further down that will tell you how to make the bread.

Ingredients

For this dish, you will need:
3 slices of gluten-free bread
4 slices of turkey ham
1 avocado
2 slices of your favorite cheese
Onion
Tomato
Canned chipotle chili peppers
Lettuce
Pickles
Alfalfa sprouts
Dijon mustard
Tabasco sauce
Light mayonnaise

Preparation:

To begin, place a skillet on the stove to heat. Once the

skillet is properly hot, place the bread on the skillet. Only toast one side of two slices of bread, but toast the third slice on both sides.

Remove the bread from the skillet, and start with one of the half-toasted slices placed toasted side down.

Onto this slice of bread, spread a bit of mayonnaise. Add 2 slices of turkey, one slice of cheese, 1 onion ring, two pickles, and the alfalfa sprouts. Sprinkle Tabasco sauce generously. Grab the fully toasted slice of bread, and spread Dijon mustard on one side and mayo on the other. Place the toast mustard side down on top of the other ingredients.

Add the last two slices of turkey onto the sandwich, along with the cheese, 1 slice of tomato, 1 diced canned chipotle pepper, 3 slices of avocado, and two leaves of lettuce. Sprinkle Tabasco sauce generously onto the sandwich, and spread Dijon mustard onto the untoasted side of the final piece of bread before completing your sandwich.

Cut in half, serve, and enjoy!

All Purpose, Gluten and Grain-Free Nut Bread

This is the nut bread that you can use to make sandwiches, cheese toast, eat with your morning coffee, or just snack on when you're hungry. It's a gluten and grain-free bread that you can use for just about anything, and it will be the perfect option regardless of what sweet or savory dish you need bread for. It's also quick and easy to make!

Ingredients:

For this dish, you will need:
¼ cup of flax meal
1 ½ cups of almond flour
Salt
4 eggs
½ teaspoon of baking soda
1 cup of walnuts, hazelnuts, almonds, and other nuts.
¼ cup of sesame seeds
¼ cup of amaranth
¼ cup of sunflower seeds
1 teaspoon of apple cider vinegar
1 teaspoon of agave honey

Preparation:

To begin, heat the oven to about 350 F, and grease two bread pans.

Combine the almond flour with the flax meal, baking

soda, and a pinch of salt in a bowl, stirring well to ensure that the ingredients are properly combined.

Crack the eggs into a bowl, and use a fork or whisk to beat them well. Make sure they are frothy, and add into the bowl the agave honey and vinegar. Mix the wet and dry ingredients together in a bowl, and add the various nuts and seeds into the same bowl. Use a fork or whisk to mix the ingredients properly until there are no lumps.

Pour the bread batter into the greased bread pans, and put them in the oven. The bread will probably take about 30 to 40 minutes to cook, so keep an eye on them. Check the bread for doneness by inserting a knife into the center, and it will come out clean when it's done cooking.

Remove from the oven, set aside to cool, and slice the bread once it has reached room temperature. You now have the ideal loaf of bread for just about anything!

Pad Thai

Pad Thai is one of the most popular Thai dishes in the country, and it will be a wonderful grain-free alternative to the more popular Chinese and Japanese fried noodle dishes. It's fairly easy to make, and it's absolutely delicious!

Ingredients

For this dish, you will need:
6 ounces of rice noodles
Sesame oil
1 onion
1 head of broccoli
Water
4 cloves of garlic
Scallions
Cilantro
Peanuts
Salt and pepper, to taste

Preparation:

To begin, place a pot of water on the stove to boil. Bring the water to a boil, and drop the rice noodles in to cook. The package will usually have clear instructions on how to cook the noodles, so follow them precisely for al dente noodles. Drain the noodles, run cold water over them, and set them aside.

Place a skillet on the stove to heat, and add a bit of sesame oil into the bottom. Dice the onion very fine, and add it into the pan to be sautéed. Cook the onions on medium-low heat, and make sure they are nicely browned.

As the onions are cooking, cut the broccoli into bite-sized spears. Once about 10 minutes has passed, add the broccoli in with the browned onions. Add ¼ cup of water, and cover the pan. Let the broccoli sauté with the onions for roughly 5 minutes, after which time it will become soft and turn a bright color.

Add salt to the pan, and dice the garlic to be added as well. Add a bit more sesame oil to ensure that the ingredients don't dry out, and add some diced peanuts into the pan. Use a tablespoon of arrowroot powder and water to thicken the mixture, and stir fry the ingredients to ensure that the powder is spread all around.

Place the noodles onto a plate, and pour the vegetable mixture over the top. If you want to add some protein, throw some shrimp into a pan and grill them to serve on top of the vegetables and noodles.

Garnish with some scallions and diced cilantro, and enjoy!

Gluten-Free Chicken Noodle Soup

There's nothing like a cup of chicken noodle soup when you're feeling ill, but wheat noodles would just make the problem worse. With this grain-free chicken noodle soup, you'll always feel better, and it is a tasty soup that you can't help but love!

Ingredients:

For this dish, you will need:
1 liter of chicken broth
1 stalk of celery
1 onions
3 cloves of garlic
1 carrot
1 zucchini
1 pack of gluten-free noodles
½ chicken breast

Preparation:

To begin, dice the onions and the carrots very finely. Make sure that they are diced very small.

Place a pot on the stove to heat, and drop a tablespoon of olive oil into the bottom. Add the garlic and onions into the pot, and sauté them until they are browned.

Once the onions and garlic are properly cooked, add the chicken broth into the pot. Set the heat on medium, and let the broth boil.

As the broth is heating up, cut the carrots into small pieces about as large as your fingernails. Throw them into the pot, along with the celery - which you will slice into small pieces as well.

Run the zucchini through a julienne slicer, and you'll have what looks like simple noodles. Put them into the pot, and let them cook along with the other ingredients.

On the side, add a bit of butter into a skillet. Slice the chicken breast into small chunks, and cook the chicken in the pot until browned on the outside. Add the partially cooked chicken into the pot of soup, ensuring that you get all the liquid and oil from the skillet.

Turn the soup up to high heat, and let it cook for another 15 minutes. Once that time has passed, drop the gluten-free soup noodles into the mixture, and let them cook on low heat. Once the noodles have cooked properly, turn off the fire and remove the pot from the stove.

Serve, add a splash of lime, and enjoy!

Gluten-Free Potato Beef Stew

Want to make a thick, hearty stew without adding flour or wheat to the mixture? This delicious stew will be an ideal meal to have on a cold winter evening, and it will be just as rich and hearty as any stew made with flour to thicken it!

Ingredients:

For this dish, you will need:
4 potatoes
1 pound of stew meat
2 carrots
1 onion
5 cloves of garlic
½ cup of table wine
¼ cup of soy sauce
1 cup of milk
2 liters of beef broth
Salt and pepper, to taste
Preparations:

To begin, peel one potato, dice it, and place it in a small pot of water to boil. Let the potato cook for about an hour, adding more water into the pot whenever necessary. Once the potato has cooked for the prescribed 60 minutes, drain all but the final dregs of water, mash with a fork, and set aside.

Place a soup pot on the stove to heat, along with a

couple of tablespoons of peanut oil in the bottom of the pot.

Dice the onion and the garlic, and add them into the pot to sauté. Add the onions first, and let them cook until nearly browned before adding in the garlic.

Dice the stew meat into small bite-sized pieces, and add them into the pot once the garlic has been properly cooked. Cook the meat until it has been browned on the outside, and add the beef broth into the pot. Bring the beef broth to a boil as you cut the other vegetables.

Cut the potatoes into medium-sized cubes, and add them into the pot. Peel and cut the potatoes into slices, and add them into the pot.

Let the stew boil for about 20 minutes, or until you're sure the potatoes are nearly cooked. Add in the soy sauce, table wine, and the milk, and let it keep cooking. Add salt and pepper as desired, along with crushed bay leaves for added flavor.

Just 5 minutes before you are about to turn the soup off, add in the mashed potato. Stir the soup well, ensuring that the mashed potato is diluted properly. The starch from the potato will thicken the stew, but it will ensure that the other ingredients aren't overcooked.

Serve with nut bread, and enjoy!

Grain-Free Ideal Breakfast

The ideal way to start the day is with a rich breakfast, but the average breakfast consists of grain-laden toast, pancakes, or other things that are made with grain. If you want the perfect breakfast without adding grain to your diet, this is the recipe for you!

Ingredients:

For this dish, you will need:
3 eggs
2 slices of turkey or Canadian bacon
6 oranges
2 Slices of Nut bread (see recipe above)
Butter
Honey
Coffee

Preparation:

To begin, place a skillet on the stove to heat. Once the skillet is hot, add the bacon and cook until done. Remove the bacon from the stove, and place on a paper towel to drain.

Leaving the bacon grease in the bottom of the pan, let it reheat until ready for the eggs. Crack one egg into the pan, and crack the other two eggs into a cup -- making sure to get only the egg whites. Add the two egg whites into the pan, and cook the eggs until done as desired. (If

you don't like your eggs to be liquid on the top, flip them over and let them sit in the pan for 3 seconds before scooping them onto your plate.)
Add the slices of nut bread onto the plate, along with the Canadian or turkey bacon. Spread butter and honey as desired on the bread, and serve yourself a cup of coffee.

Squeeze the oranges, and enjoy your fresh cup of OJ for the ideal grain-free breakfast!

Dark Chicken Soup

If you're not too particular about the way your soup looks, you'll find that this will be the ideal meal for you! It comes loaded with all the nutrients you need, and there are even a few noodles floating around to help fill you up. All in all, however, it's a nicely low calorie meal - and grain-free as well!

Ingredients

For this dish, you will need:
2 liters of chicken broth
1 bunch of chard
2 carrots
1 bunch of spinach
1 cup of shitake mushrooms
1 pack of shitake mushroom noodles
¼ pound of chicken breast

Preparation:

To begin, place the chard and spinach in a pot with 2 cups of water and 2 cups of chicken stock. Bring the veggies to a boil, and let them cook until they are soft. Pour the soup into the food processor, blend it until it is completely liquefied, and set it aside.

Pour the chicken broth into a pot, and bring it to a boil. Cut the carrots and shitake mushrooms into slices, and add them into the soup. Pour the liquefied dark greens into the pot, and let them cook along with the chicken broth.

In a pan on the side, add a pat of butter into the bottom as the pan heats. Dice the chicken breast into chunks, and let the breast cook until it is browned on the outside. Once it is nearly cooked, pour the chicken and the grease into the soup pot. Let it cook until you're sure the chicken is thoroughly done.

Add the mushroom noodles a few minutes before you want to cook the soup, and follow the cooking instructions on the package. The noodles shouldn't take too long to cook, and you can serve out the soup while it's still piping hot!

Carrot Muffins

These delicious muffins will help you to start the day out right, and you can munch on a couple of them as you head to work. Thanks to the fact that they're completely grain-free, they'll be the perfect option for you!

Ingredients

For this dish, you will need:
¼ teaspoon of baking soda
¼ cup of coconut flour
Cinnamon
3 eggs
Salt
¼ cup of oil
¼ cup of natural molasses
Vanilla
3 carrots
¼ cup of raspberries, blackberries, and black currants

Preparation:

To begin, preheat the oven to about 350 F. This is the perfect temperature for muffins, as it will keep cooking time down without risking burning the muffins.

Combine the baking soda, coconut flour, and a teaspoon of cinnamon in a bowl, and stir it well to ensure that it's properly combined.

In a separate bowl, crack and mix the eggs. Whip them until they are frothy, and pour the oil, molasses, and a teaspoon of vanilla into the mix. Beat well, add a pinch of salt, and combine the wet ingredients with the dry.

Use a whisk to combine the wet and dry ingredients well, and stir until you are sure there are no lumps.

With a bit of butter, grease a muffin tray. You'll get about 12 to 18 medium-sized muffins, though as many as 30 mini muffins. Put the tray into the oven, and cook the muffins for about 30 minutes. Insert a knife into the top of one muffin, and it should come out clean once it's done.

Remove the muffins from the oven, scoop them out of their tray, and set them aside to cool.

Almond and Grilled Chicken Salad

The beauty of salads is that they are some of the best grain-free recipes, and you won't have to worry about getting gluten if you eat a healthy salad. If you want to really go all out with the salad, add nuts and lots of filling veggies! You'll find that it will be tasty and very enjoyable!

Ingredients:

For this dish, you will need:
1 pound of chicken breast
1 head of Romaine or Iceberg lettuce
1 cup of raw almonds
1 cup of raw peanuts
1 cup of dried cranberries
1 apple
½ cup of olive oil
½ cup of apple cider vinegar
1 cup of gluten-free soy sauce
Salt
Sesame seeds

Preparation:

To begin, slice the chicken breast into steaks about ¾ inch thick. You'll get about 3 steaks from a single chicken breast. Place the chicken breast on a grill, and rub a seasoning of salt, pepper, garlic, and Parmesan cheese onto the breast before cooking it. Grill the chicken well on both sides, and make sure that the middle of the chicken is cooked before removing it from the grill. Set the chicken aside.

Soak the lettuce in a bowl of ice cold water, which will make it crunchy and crispy. Once the lettuce has soaked for 30 minutes, use your hands to rip it into bite-sized leaves.

Slice the apple into quarters, cut out the cores, and cut the apple into small chunks. Add the apples into the salad, along with the cranberries.

In a skillet on the stove, place the almonds and peanuts together. The raw nuts will need to be toasted, and they will take about 20 minutes. Make sure to stir them every 5 minutes or so, and keep the heat on medium high to prevent them from burning. Once the almonds and peanuts are toasted, add them into the salad.

Slice the chicken breast into strips, and add them into the salad as well.

Combine the vinegar, soy sauce, and olive oil together, along with a pinch of salt and some black pepper. Pour this mixture over the salad, and sprinkle sesame seeds liberally on top to garnish the salad. It's now ready for you to eat!

Gluten-Free Breakfast Biscuits

There's nothing like a delicious, buttery biscuit to start your day off on the right foot, and these grain-free biscuits will be just what you need to enjoy your morning. They're easy to whip up, and you can take them with you to snack in your car on the way to work.

Ingredients

For this dish, you will need:
2 cups of almond flour
½ teaspoon of baking soda
2 eggs
1 teaspoon of honey
1/3 cup of butter or margarine
Salt

Preparation:

To begin, preheat the oven to about 350 F. This is the temperature that will allow the biscuits to turn golden brown on the outside, but without making the center of the biscuits too dry.

In a bowl, combine the almond flour with the baking soda and a pinch of salt. Stir well to ensure that there are no clumps of baking soda.

In another bowl, crack the eggs and beat them until they are frothy. Add in the butter and the honey, and beat well. You'll want to keep stirring until you have a slightly creamy mixture.

Fold the wet ingredients gently into the dry ones, and mix until you're sure that there are no lumps. You will need to keep stirring as the dough is formed.

Use a piece of greased baking paper to roll the biscuit dough out, and keep rolling until you've flattened the dough to about 1 ½ inches thick. Use a jar with a wide mouth to cut out the biscuits, and keep rolling the dough until you have turned it all into biscuits.

Transfer the biscuits to an oven tray with a piece of greased baking paper, and put the tray into the oven. Let the biscuits cook for about 15 minutes, and keep a close eye on them. You'll notice that the rounded edges of the biscuits will start to brown, and don't let them get too dark before removing them from the oven.

Use a spatula to scrape the biscuits off the greased baking sheet, and set them on a rack to cool. Once they're cool, spread a bit of butter and honey on them, and enjoy!

Nutty Granola

Granola is one of the best breakfasts that you can have, and you'll find that this nutty granola will be just the thing to stoke up your internal furnace first thing in the morning. It's a grain-free breakfast that will kick off your day in style!

Ingredients

For this dish, you will need:
1 cup of steel cut oats
2 cups of almonds
1 cup of amaranth
1 cup of raisins
1 cup of walnuts
1 tablespoon of vanilla
Butter
Cinnamon
Sugar

Preparation:

To begin, place a skillet on the stove to heat. Melt a cup of butter in the bottom of the skillet, and add the oats in once the butter is liquefied completely.

Use a spatula or wooden spoon to roll the oats thoroughly in the butter, and ensure that the oats are properly coated. Remove the skillet from the heat, and transfer the oats into a flat baking tray.

Preheat the oven to 350 F.

Add the raisins into the oats, and cut the almonds and walnuts in half. Add in the amaranth, and sprinkle a bit of sugar, cinnamon, and a few tablespoons of vanilla extract onto the oats. Make sure that the oats are mixed properly, and put the tray into the oven to cook.

Give the oats about 30 minutes to cook at 350 F, but keep checking them to ensure that they don't burn. You'll find that they'll become nice and crunchy once they've cooked properly, but let them cool down before eating them.

Grain-Free Breakfast Bars

Need something quick to munch on as you drive to work in the morning? Don't let the heavy traffic get you down, but make these delicious breakfast bars to help keep your mind off the fact that you're sitting and doing nothing. They're a healthy breakfast that you can enjoy on the go!

Ingredients

For this dish, you will need:
2 cups of almond flour
1/3 teaspoon of baking soda
1/3 cup of grapeseed oil
Vanilla extract
1/3 cup of honey
½ cup of shredded coconut
1/3 cup of raisins
1/3 cup of nuts (your preference)
¼ cup of flax seeds
¼ cup of amaranth
¼ pumpkin seeds

Preparation:

To begin, preheat the oven to 350 F.

In a bowl, combine the almond flour with a pinch of salt and the baking soda. Make sure to mix well, as that will eliminate any lumps of baking soda.

In another bowl, mix the honey with a tablespoon of vanilla and the grapeseed oil. The oil will be a bit hard to mix in, but a bit of effort will yield a properly mixed liquid.

Pour the wet ingredients in with the dry ones, and whisk vigorously to ensure that the wet and dry ingredients combine nicely without any lumps.

Once you're done mixing, add the nuts, seeds, raisins, coconut, and amaranth into the batter. Mix well to distribute the latest additions.

Use a bit of butter to grease the bottom of a baking tray, and pour the mixture into the pan. Place the pan in the oven, and let it cook for about 20 minutes at 350 F. You'll find that it turns a nice golden brown, and it will become very crunchy and a bit hard to cut.

Slice the bars into small pieces, and serve or set aside to eat on the go.

Garden-Style Hot Dogs

Hot dogs are one of the most popular American foods around, but the problem is the hot dog bun. If you want to enjoy a classic hot dog in a very unique way, these garden-style hot dogs will be an ideal way for you to eliminate the gluten from your meal.

Ingredients:

For this dish, you will need:
6 hot dogs
6 slices of bacon
1 head of Romaine lettuce
½ tomato
½ onion
Pickle relish
Sauerkraut
Ketchup
Mayo
Mustard
Tabasco sauce

Preparation:

To begin, soak the head of lettuce in ice cold water. The cold water will help to make the lettuce crunchier and crispier, which will make it much easier to eat.

Place a skillet on the stove, and let it heat. As the pan is heating, wrap one strip of bacon around each hotdog.

You can hold the bacon in place using toothpicks, but make sure that the toothpicks don't interfere with the cooking process.

Let the hot dogs cook for about 20 minutes on low heat, and turn them regularly to ensure that they don't burn. The grease from the bacon will make them very tasty.

Once they're thoroughly cooked, remove the skillet from the stove, but leave the hot dogs inside.

Remove 12 strips of lettuce, and make 6 stacks of two leaves. Dice the tomato and the onions, making sure that they are very small.

Place a bit of sauerkraut in **the bottom** layer of lettuce, and stack the second leaf on top. Place each hot dog into the top leaf, and add tomato, onion, and pickle relish on top. Add the condiments of your choice, and enjoy the delicious, all-natural hot dog meal!

Grain-Free Mac and Cheese

Mac and Cheese is the quintessential American meal, but egg noodles are made with wheat. Using gluten-free noodles will allow you to still enjoy this delicious dish, but without having to worry about adding grain to your meal!

Ingredients

For this dish, you will need:
2 packs of gluten-free noodles
3 cups of grated cheddar cheese
½ cup of butter
1 ½ cups of milk
2 tablespoons of heavy cream
¼ pound of bacon
1 onion
4 cloves of garlic

Preparation:

To begin, place a skillet on the stove to heat. Add a bit of butter into the bottom of the skillet, and dice the onions as the pan gets hot. Add the onions into the bottom of the pan to sauté, and dice the garlic to add in once the onions begin to brown.

Remove the garlic and onions from the stove once the aroma of the garlic is extracted, and slice the bacon as the skillet heats up once again. Place a pot of water on the stove to boil, which will be for the noodles.

Once the skillet is hot, add the bacon into the pan. Cook until it is nicely browned, and remove from the stove.

Place the onions and garlic back on the stove, and pour the milk and bacon into the pan. Once the milk gets hot, add in the heavy cream and the butter. Bring the ingredients to a boil, and add the cheddar cheese into the mix. Turn the fire off, but leave the pan on the stove.

Boil the noodles, and cook them until they are al dente. Place the noodles back into the pot they were cooked in, add the cheese sauce over the top, garnish with a bit more cheese, and serve while hot!

Almond Raisin Muffins

These muffins are simple and easy to make, but they'll be delicious without a doubt! You can even top them with icing to make delicious cupcakes, or keep them light if you're on a diet! Enjoy them no matter where you are, as they are fantastic.

Ingredients:

For this dish, you will need:
1 cup of flax meal
1 cup of almond flour
1 tablespoon of baking powder
Nutmeg
Cinnamon
½ cup of raisins
1/3 cup of toasted **almonds**
1 stick of butter
Salt
4 eggs
½ cup of sugar
½ cup of buttermilk
2 tablespoons of brown sugar

Preparation:

To begin, you will need to heat the oven to about 375 F. Once the oven is hot, turn it down to 350 F, which is the ideal temperature for baking the muffins.

Combine the baking powder, flax meal, almond flour, and a pinch of salt in a bowl, mixing well to combine. Add a teaspoon each of cinnamon and nutmeg, and stir well.

Combine the butter, eggs, sugar, and milk in a bowl, and beat until the eggs are frothy and the butter is creamy. Using melted butter will make the process a lot quicker, but you can use an egg beater if you don't want to take the time to melt the butter.

Combine the wet and dry ingredients, and mix them well to eliminate any lumps. Add the raisins into the mix. Chop the toasted almonds into small pieces, and add them into the muffin batter as well.

Once the ingredients are all stirred in well, pour the muffin batter into a muffin baking tray. Use paper muffin cups if you want to limit the mess.

Place the muffins in the oven, and let them cook for roughly 15 to 20 minutes, depending the altitude of your city(it takes longer for things to bake the higher above sea level you are). Insert a toothpick into the top of the muffins when they look cooked, and they are done when the toothpick comes out clean.

Remove the muffins from the tray, set them aside to cool, and serve.

Grain-Free Pizza

Pizza is one of the most popular dishes in the world, but it's hard to make a good pizza without using flour. This pizza is made without wheat, and it's a tasty alternative that gluten-sensitive people can enjoy without worrying about their stomachs acting up.

Ingredients

For this dish, you will need:

1 cup of quinoa flour
1 cup of potato flour
1 cup of almond flour
1 cup of buckwheat
Salt
Xantham gum
4 teaspoons of dried yeast
Canola or olive oil
Water
Tomato sauce
Cheese
Pizza toppings of your choice

Preparation:

To begin, heat the oven to a toasty 350 F.

Grease some baking sheets with a bit of olive or canola oil, and place them on the trays where you will be cooking your pizza.

Sift the various flours, salt, and baking soda into a bowl, and combine the dry ingredients well. Add the yeast into the mixture.

Mix half a liter of warm water with a couple of tablespoons of olive oil, and add the wet ingredients into the dry ones. Mix the dough until it is properly combined, and set it aside for a few minutes to rise.

Once it has risen, use a spoon to scoop it into your pizza tray. Make a nicely rounded pizza, and put it in the oven to cook until the crust is golden brown.

All that is left to do is to scoop the pizza or tomato sauce onto the top of the crust, add cheese, and top with the ingredients of your choice. Put the crust back into the oven, and cook it until the cheese has properly melted.

Slice, serve, and enjoy!

Your Grain Free Meal Plan

So, you've got all these awesome grain-free recipes to work with! Whether you're trying to lose weight or just stay healthy, eating these foods will help you to keep grain and gluten out of your life. If you want to add these delicious meals to your diet, here is an 11-day meal plan that you can use to incorporate all of these recipes into your life:

Day 1:
Breakfast: Buckwheat Pancakes
Lunch: Eggs and Nut Bread Toast
Dinner: Pad Thai

Day 2:
Breakfast: Gluten Free Waffles
Lunch: Grain-Free Cornbread with Grilled Chicken or Steak, plus plenty of veggies
Dinner: Special K cereal (made with rice rather than wheat flour)

Day 3:
Breakfast: Special K Cereal
Lunch: Stuffed Bell Peppers
Dinner: Chicken with Rice Stuffing
Dessert: Roasted Almond Cookies

Day 4:
Breakfast: Apple Cobbler

Lunch: Asian Sesame Noodles
Dinner: Almond and Grilled Chicken Salad

Day 5:
Breakfast: Breakfast Cereal Sans Gluten
Lunch: Grain Free Breaded Chicken with Nut Bread and veggies
Dinner: Gluten-Free Chicken Noodle Soup with Nut Bread
Dessert: Gluten and Sugar-Free Gingerbread Cake

Day 6:
Breakfast: Carrot Muffins
Lunch: Gluten-Free Turkey Club
Dinner: Curried Quinoa with Chick Peas

Day 7:
Breakfast: Grain-Free Ideal Breakfast
Lunch: Dark Chicken Soup with Nut Bread
Dinner: Grain-Free Mac and Cheese

Day 8:
Breakfast: Gluten-Free Breakfast Biscuits
Lunch: Gluten-Free Potato Beef Stew
Dinner: Shrimp Cakes
Dessert: Gluten-Free Irish Shortbread

Day 9:
Breakfast: Nutty Granola
Lunch: Dark Chicken Soup with Nut Bread
Dinner: Special K Cereal

Day 10:
Breakfast: Breakfast Bars
Lunch: Garden-Style Hot Dogs
Dinner: Sesame Seed Chicken Fried Steak

Day 11:
Breakfast: Almond Flour Muffins
Lunch: Grain-Free Pizza
Dinner: Special K Cereal

The meal plan above doesn't come with the calorie count on each food item, but that's something that won't be as important as the fact that they are all grain-free foods. You can eat them without worrying too much about calories, but try and keep the consumption of these foods to a healthy minimum in order to avoid gaining weight!

All of these recipes can be found online, though some of them are our own original creations. You can probably find similar recipes on websites like AllRecpes.com, About.com, and particularly ElanasPantry.com. They are all recipes that someone made, and we just wanted to share them with you. We've made a few adjustments to the various recipes so that you'll get only our unique grain-free flavor on the recipes, but you'll find that there are many like them. The important thing is that you can enjoy your grain-free cooking and eating, and we wanted to provide you with a recipe book that you can use to prepare delicious meals free of grain and gluten.

We apologize if you've seen these recipes elsewhere, and we hope that you enjoy the creations we have presented to you!

[1] http://www.stuff.co.nz/life-style/38883/The-effects-of-gluten-on-health

www.ingramcontent.com/pod-product-compliance
Ingram Content Group UK Ltd.
Pitfield, Milton Keynes, MK11 3LW, UK
UKHW020654080426
11746UKWH00032B/633

9 781631 878886